Diabetic Complications

Diabetic Complications

Edited by

K. M. SHAW

Department of Diabetes and Endocrinology,
Queen Alexandra Hospital, Portsmouth, UK

John Wiley & Sons

Chichester · New York · Brisbane · Toronto · Singapore

Other Wiley Editorial Offices

John Wiley & Sons, Inc., 605 Third Avenue,
New York, NY 10158-0012, USA

Jacaranda Wiley Ltd, 33 Park Road, Milton,
Queensland 4064, Australia

John Wiley & Sons (Canada) Ltd, 22 Worcester Road,
Rexdale, Ontario M9W 1L1, Canada

John Wiley & Sons (Asia) Pte Ltd, 2 Clementi Loop #02-01,
Jin Xing Distripark, Singapore 0512

Library of Congress Cataloging-in-Publication Data

Diabetic complications / edited by K. Shaw.
    p.   cm. – (Practical diabetes series)
    Includes bibliographical references and index.
    ISBN 0-471-96678-9 (hbk : alk. paper)
    1. Diabetes—Complications.   I. Shaw, K. (Kenneth)   II. Series:
Practical diabetes (Chichester, England)
    [DNLM: 1. Diabetes Mellitus—complications.   WK 835 D53492 1996]
RC660.D5836   1996
616.4′62—dc20
DNLM/DLC
for Library of Congress   96-10648
                                                              CIP

British Library Cataloguing in Publication Data

A catalogue record for this book is available from the British Library

ISBN 0-471-96678-9

Typeset in 10/12pt Palatino by Acorn Bookwork, Salisbury, Wiltshire
Printed and bound in Great Britain by Biddles, Guildford
This book is printed on acid-free paper responsibly manufactured from sustainable
forestation, for which at least two trees are planted for each one used for paper production.

Contents

List of Contributors

Dr W. ALEXANDER   *Consultant Physician, Diabetes Unit, Queen Mary's Hospital, Sidcup, Kent DA14 6LT*

Dr D. BOASE   *Consultant Opthalmologist, Eye Department, Queen Alexandra Hospital, Cosham, Portsmouth PO6 3LY*

Professor D. G. COLIN-JONES   *Consultant Physician and Professor of Gastroenterology, Queen Alexandra Hospital, Cosham, Portsmouth PO6 3LY*

Ms S. CRADOCK, Ms A. TIER and Ms J. WOOD   *Diabetes Specialist Nurses, Queen Alexandra Hospital, Cosham, Portsmouth PO6 3LY*

Dr M. CUMMINGS   *Consultant Physician, Department of Diabetes and Endocrinology, Queen Alexandra Hospital, Cosham, Portsmouth PO6 3LY*

Dr M. EDMONDS   *Diabetic Department, Kings College Hospital, Denmark Hill, London SE5 9RS*

Dr A. V. M. FOSTER   *Diabetic Department, Kings College Hospital, Denmark Hill, London SE5 9RS*

Dr C. J. HEAVEN   *Senior Registrar, Manchester Royal Eye Hospital, Oxford Road, Manchester M13 9WH*

Dr A. MACLEOD   *Consultant Physician, Royal Shrewsbury Hospital, Mytton Oak Road, Shrewsbury SY3 8XQ*

Dr G. VENKAT RAMAN   *Consultant Physician, Wessex Renal and Transplant Unit, University of Southampton, St Mary's Hospital, Milton Road, Portsmouth PO3 6AD*

Professor K. M. SHAW	*Consultant Physician, Department of Diabetes and Endocrinology, Queen Alexandra Hospital, Cosham, Portsmouth PO6 3LY and Visiting Professor, University of Portsmouth*
Professor P. SÖNKSEN	*Professor of Endocrinology, Department of Endocrinology and Chemical Pathology, St Thomas' Hospital, Lambeth Palace Road, London SE1 7EH*
Dr P. J. WATKINS	*Consultant Physician, Diabetic Department, King's College Hospital, Denmark Hill, London SE5 9RS*
Dr G. F. WATTS	*Senior Lecturer and Consultant Physician, University Department of Medicine, Royal Perth Hospital, Medical Research Foundation Building, Level 4, Rear 50 Murray Street, Perth WA 6000, Australia*

Preface

We appear to be on the threshold of witnessing a substantial reduction in the long-term complications of diabetes. Modern treatment regimens, better monitoring of control and the huge impact of improved education all combine to offer the prospect of real progress towards prevention of complications and lessening of progression in those in whom complications may be present. The Diabetes Control and Complications Trial (DCCT) has provided evidence that such can be achieved, while the St Vincent Declaration initiative has set the standards to enable these benefits to become reality.

Such is the encouraging future expectation that the logistics of delivering the necessary diabetes care to achieve the potential immense health gain are still daunting. Much more diabetes care is being undertaken in general practice as structured mini-clinics are established, while hospital diabetes centres have never been busier as more specialized complex cases are referred. Never has organized multi-professional teamwork across all sectors of health care been needed more. Whether the patient is managed at a hospital centre, in a community mini-clinic or on a shared-care basis, the importance of identifying those patients at risk of complications and the detection of developing complications at an early stage is now beyond dispute.

The contributors to this book have extensive experience in diabetes, either as specialists specifically in diabetes or as experts in other fields to whom complications of diabetes are referred. Each contribution seeks to outline the nature of diabetes complications, how susceptibility and risk can be identified, the importance of screening during the early stages and the way appropriate investigation and management should be undertaken.

It is hoped that those of all disciplines involved in the day-to-day care and education of diabetes, either in the community or in the specialist centre, will find both interest and practical help from the content of this book. The St Vincent's objective of reducing and even eliminating complications of diabetes is now a real and achievable goal.

K. M. Shaw
Portsmouth, February 1996

Foreword

Nearly three-quarters of a century has passed since the discovery of insulin, and while there is scarcely anyone who can now recall diabetes treatment before 1922, there are many whose memories extend over 60 years or more to the early exhilarating era of insulin treatment. Some recall their physicians of the time, notably perhaps Dr R. D. Lawrence of King's College Hospital, that flamboyant, yet astute and most caring of physicians. Yet those with long memories and long lives have survived a life of diabetes, happily spared the development of diabetic complications. The absence of complications may have been due in part to good management, but a genetic influence is probably as important.

The euphoria of the 1920s was followed by recognition of most of the disorders due to diabetic complications in the following decades. Yet by mid-century physicians could only observe the outcome with little chance of having any influence on the natural progression of the disease. Nephropathy and retinopathy frequently led to renal failure and blindness while the consequences of neuropathy and vascular disease resulted in catastrophic foot disease and amputations.

In the last 25 years there has been a dramatic change. The benefits of tight metabolic control have been demonstrated in numerous studies, most recently and most conclusively in the Diabetes Control and Complications Trial (DCCT) in the USA. It is now possible to reduce the incidence of complications by 35–70%, or when they occur to retard their progression. This magnificent study gives enormous encouragement to both patients and their physicians and nurses by demonstrating that their efforts are really worth while. It gives renewed impetus to the search for achieving better diabetes control without developing the devastating consequences of hypoglycaemia.

Extraordinary developments have also evolved in treating the consequences of diabetic complications when they do occur. In Germany, photocoagulation was used empirically to prevent the evolution of retinopathy and was subsequently shown to prevent blindness. The evolution of nephropathy can be substantially reduced by hypotensive treatment, and the potential specific advantage of angiotensin-converting enzyme inhibitors has been demonstrated. Dialysis and transplantation are now available to most diabetic patients who need renal support treatment, although even a decade ago, many centres considered that diabetic patients did not qualify for these treatments. The availability especially of continuous ambulatory peritoneal dialysis (CAPD) has transformed the availability of renal support even in elderly patients who can achieve a very acceptable quality of life. Treatment of the diabetic foot has been revolutionized: primary prevention of foot ulcers by education, chiropody and advice on footwear represents probably the best and most cost-effective prevention measure in the care of diabetic patients. The establishment of specialized foot clinics leads to rapid treatment of threatening lesions, and amputation rate can thereby be halved. Angioplasty and vascular surgery have advanced to the point where they make an important contribution to limb salvage.

Proper care in the 1990s must therefore include the facilities for identification of all patients with diabetes—hence the need for diabetes registers—and the regular review for early detection of complications which will enable physicians to take the steps needed to abort the disease. These requirements place a huge demand on society in terms of health resources, but the demands of our patients are now heard, and governments have acknowledged the need to reduce complications following wide acceptance of the St Vincent declaration. So it is the organization of diabetes care which must change to accommodate these developments. The introduction of the diabetes specialist nurse is probably the most important innovation in diabetes care, and his/her expertise now enables delivery of care on a community basis, linked of course to the strength of diabetes expertise and research at the hospital-based diabetes departments. These new arrangements must be made to achieve high standards, and there should be a new era of optimism which might lead to a reduction of the tragedies of diabetes, just as improved standards reduced fetal mortality from over 30% in the 1940s to between 1 and 2% in the 1990s.

This book addresses these topical issues in a comprehensive approach, and describes in detail methods for early detection of diabetes complications by the extended team ranging from the community base to the hospital. Specialist nurses are responsible for one of the chapters giving an indication of their key role not just in the care of patients, but also in the organization of screening and education programmes, now crucial to the provision of high-quality diabetes care.

There can be few fields in medicine in which such important advances have been made in little more than two decades. As the British Diabetic Association, which has done so much to advance understanding of the disease and help public understanding of its needs, celebrates its 60th birthday, both those with diabetes and those who care for them should have a renewed optimism for the future. The advances stem, of course, from the events in 1922 when the earliest patients were treated with insulin, and Elizabeth Hughes wrote to her mother that 'Dr Banting considers my progress simply miraculous'. The advances continue to this day.

P. J. Watkins
Diabetic Department
King's College Hospital
London

1

Diabetic Retinopathy

C. J. HEAVEN and D. L. BOASE*

Manchester Royal Eye Hospital, Manchester and
*Eye Department, Queen Alexandra Hospital, Portsmouth

INTRODUCTION

Despite the advent of retinal laser photocoagulation, and more recently vitreoretinal surgery, diabetic retinopathy remains a blinding disorder. Indeed in recent decades it has been the commonest cause of blind registration amongst those of working age in the UK[1,2]. It has yet to be shown whether, in the face of the increasing prevalence of diabetes, these modern treatment modalities have altered this situation or not.

The main causes of visual loss from diabetic retinopathy are disturbance to the macula, affecting central vision (diabetic maculopathy), and profound retinal ischaemia leading to proliferative retinopathy. The risk of developing diabetic retinopathy increases with the duration of the diabetes. At diagnosis less than 5% of patients will have retinopathy. After 10 years the prevalence rises to 40–50%, and after 20 years more than 90% of patients will have some form of retinal abnormality[3]. When these changes threaten vision, early treatment can prevent sight loss in many cases. However, late presentation and the as yet untreatable forms of diabetic retinopathy continue to present a major challenge in terms of prevention and alleviation of blindness.

PATHOGENESIS

A basic grasp of retinal anatomy is helpful in understanding the aetiology of diabetic retinopathy, its classification and the modes of treatment and their consequences.

Diabetic Complications. Edited by K. M. Shaw
© 1996 John Wiley & Sons Ltd

The optic disc is the most readily identifiable feature of the ocular fundus. It is located approximately 15 degrees nasal to the visual axis and is the channel through which the retinal nerve fibres leave the eye to form the optic nerve. The central retinal artery and vein also enter and leave the eye at this point, respectively. There are no photoreceptors (rods and cones) at the optic disc which corresponds to the blind spot of vision. The macula is that area of the retina bounded by the optic disc and the temporal superior and inferior main vascular arcades. This is approximately equivalent to the histological definition of the macula as the area of the retina where the ganglion cell layer is more than one cell thick. The macula is responsible for the central 20 to 30 degrees of vision. The fovea is the area of retina (approximately disc sized) located at the centre of the macula and is responsible for the fine visual acuity characteristic of the central 5 degrees of vision.

The retina has a complex multilayered structure of photoreceptors and nerve cells. It is inverted in the sense that the photoreceptors lie deepest in proximity to the pigment epithelium and choroid. The neural elements overlie the photoreceptors with the nerve fibre layer (axons of the ganglion cells) on the anterior surface adjacent to the vitreous. Light entering the eye must therefore pass through the substance of the retina before being detected by the photoreceptors. This degrades image clarity. To overcome this problem, at the fovea the layers of nerve cells are swept to the side to facilitate direct access of light to the photoreceptors (Figure 1.1). The retina at this location is consequently thin and crater like. This specialization at the fovea leaves it particularly vulnerable to certain forms of diabetic maculopathy.

The health and high metabolic activity of the retina depends upon the retinal capillary bed. This capillary bed extends net-like throughout the retina except for a small area at the very centre of the macula known as the 'foveal avascular zone'. The fundamental defect in all forms of diabetic retinopathy is a disturbance to these retinal capillaries. In simple terms these vessels may either become blocked and non-perfused or may leak. Blockage and non-perfusion lead to retinal ischaemia which if profound may stimulate the growth (proliferation) of retinal new vessels. Leakage may be of any of the blood constituents. Retinal haemorrhage results from leakage of erythrocytes, retinal oedema from leakage of plasma fluid and retinal exudate from leakage and deposition of plasma lipoproteins. At a microstructural level this capillary dysfunction occurs as a result of thickening and abnormal composition of the vascular basement membrane, endothelial cell damage and proliferation and loss of pericytes from the vessel wall[4]. Changes in the flow characteristics and coagulability of the blood itself may also be contributory[4].

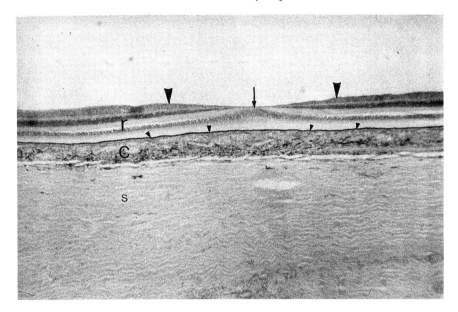

Figure 1.1. Histological section through the macula. Note the complex multi-layered structure of the retina: r = retina, c = choroid, s = sclera. The foveal crater lies between the large arrow heads. The arrow demarcates the centre of the fovea; the point of maximum visual acuity. Here the inner retinal layers are displaced centrifugally allowing more direct access of light to the photoreceptors. This anatomical specialization accounts for certain specific forms of diabetic maculopathy. The small arrow heads indicate the retinal pigment epithelium separating the retina and choroid. (Courtesy of Dr R. Bonshek, Manchester Royal Eye Hospital)

CLINICAL FEATURES OF DIABETIC RETINOPATHY

Diabetic retinopathy may be classified as follows:

- Background retinopathy
- Diabetic maculopathy
- Pre-proliferative retinopathy
- Proliferative retinopathy.

In addition, failure to quench proliferative retinopathy may result in various forms of advanced diabetic eye disease.

BACKGROUND DIABETIC RETINOPATHY

This is the mildest form of diabetic retinopathy and is not in itself vision threatening. Its characteristic feature is the retinal capillary micro-aneurysm. These saccular dilatations are thought to form in two ways. A local distension of the retinal capillary may occur due to weakness within the vessel wall, probably as a result of loss of structurally supportive peri-cytes. Alternatively microaneurysms may originate from partial fusion of the adjacent arms of capillary kinks or loops[5].

When viewed with white light microaneurysms appear as red dots. They are though more apparent when viewed using red-free light (green). This increases the contrast between the orange fundus and the red micro-aneurysms, which then appear as black dots. Fluorescein angiography usually reveals many more microaneurysms than can be seen clinically (Figure 1.2). However, this investigation is not justified for this reason alone.

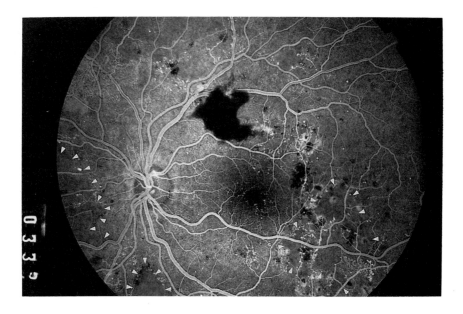

Figure 1.2. Fundus fluorescein angiogram of left eye. Arrows outline areas of capillary non-perfusion. Dark areas represent retinal haemorrhage masking fluores-cence. Note the large number of microaneurysms and the foveal avascular zone. Intraretinal microvascular abnormalities (IRMAs) are present superonasally and inferotemporally and there is also slight irregularity of the retinal veins (beading), indicating significant retinal ischaemia. (Courtesy of Mr R. E. Butler, Queen Alex-andra Hospital, Portsmouth)

The term microaneurysm should not be confused with macroaneurysm. Macroaneurysms are saccular dilatations on the retinal arterioles. Macroaneurysms are not a feature of diabetic retinopathy.

The other features of background diabetic retinopathy are small retinal haemorrhages, retinal exudate and 'cotton wool spots'. However, if these features occur within the macula the retinopathy should be classified as maculopathy rather than background.

The retinal haemorrhages of background retinopathy may occur either within the retinal substance or more superficially amongst the nerve fibre layer. When present within the retina they are confined by its structure and appear as small dots a little larger than microaneurysms. When in the nerve fibre layer they tend to form streaks of flame-shaped patterns. Typically the haemorrhages of background retinopathy are small and few in number scattered here and there throughout the fundus. Accumulations of large blotchy haemorrhages may represent a more serious form of retinopathy.

Retinal exudate has a yellow appearance with well-defined edges. It may occur as isolated flecks or in clusters which often take the form of circles known as 'circinates'. This pattern arises as a result of focal vascular leakage. Plasma fluid spreads centrifugally from the point of leakage into the surrounding retina. Lipoprotein is then deposited at the limit of this fluid rather akin to a 'high tide mark'. When present outside the macula retinal exudate does not require treatment. Usually the point of leakage eventually seals and over the course of several months the exudate resolves. Fresh circinates may meanwhile appear around new points of leakage elsewhere.

'Cotton wool spots' represent local retinal ischaemia. The term is very descriptive of their fluffy white appearance with ill-defined edges. They occur in the nerve fibre layer on the surface of the retina, obscuring its deeper structure, and are the result of a local accumulation of axoplasm. Normally the constituents within each retinal ganglion cell axon are continually moving up and down the fibre. This axoplasmic transport system is an energy-dependent active process and reliant on the integrity of the retinal capillary bed. If a bundle of nerve fibres crosses an area of retinal capillary closure the axoplasmic transport fails at that point. However, axoplasmic transport continues on either side of the lesion where the retinal capillary bed is intact. Because the axoplasm is transported in both directions simultaneously an accumulation of material occurs at the site of ischaemia.

In isolation cotton wool spots carry no worse a visual prognosis than the other features of background retinopathy. However, as part of a picture of widespread retinal ischaemia and deep blotchy haemorrhages, they may be more sinister.

Cotton wool spots used to be called soft exudates. As they do not result from vascular leakage this term has rightly been abandoned.

DIABETIC MACULOPATHY

Diabetic maculopathy accounts for the majority of blindness from diabetic retinopathy. This is due to two factors. Firstly, non-insulin-dependent diabetes is much more common than insulin-dependent diabetes. Secondly, in broad terms, maculopathy tends to be associated with older non-insulin-dependent diabetic patients whereas proliferative retinopathy tends to be associated with younger insulin-dependent diabetics[3,6].

Diabetic maculopathy may take several forms depending on the precise changes occurring within the retinal capillary bed. These forms may coexist:

- Ischaemic maculopathy

- Exudative maculopathy

- Macula oedema.

Ischaemic maculopathy results from extensive capillary closure within the central retina. The macula has a particularly high metabolic activity. In the absence of adequate perfusion visual processing fails, atrophic changes set in and visual acuity is reduced. The macula takes on a pale and featureless appearance punctuated by haemorrhage and microaneurysms. The microaneurysms tend to occur at the junction of perfused and non-perfused capillary bed. There are no exudates. This form of maculopathy is untreatable.

In diabetic maculopathy vascular leakage may be either focal or diffuse. An exudative maculopathy occurs with focal leakage. Escaping plasma lipoproteins may cause hard exudate formation as in background retinopathy. However, the exudate formation differs in two respects from that outside the macula. It may be vision threatening, the more so the nearer it is to the fovea, and the pattern of exudate formation is dictated by the peculiar anatomy of the macula. In the periphery of the macula, adjacent to the temporal vascular arcades, circinate exudates are produced as in background retinopathy (Figure 1.3). However, when the leakage point is nearer to the fovea the plasma fluid will tend to run down the sides of the foveal crater depositing exudate amongst Henle's fibres. This results in the formation of radiating spokes of hard exudate which may accumulate to form a partial or even complete macula star with the fovea at its centre (Figure 1.4). Hard exudate within the retina disrupts its microanatomy and function. This is especially true at the fovea where the retina is thin and relatively poorly compacted. Laser treatment should therefore be given

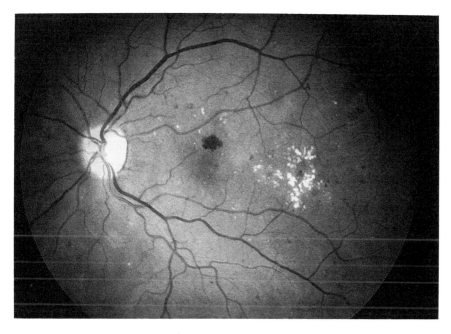

Figure 1.3. Exudative diabetic maculopathy of left eye. Hard exudate in the form of several small overlapping 'circinates' is present in the temporal macula. The fovea, and visual acuity, are not immediately threatened but focal laser treatment is required. This will seal the causative local vascular leakage, allow absorption of the exudate and prevent visual deterioration

early in exudative maculopathy before irreversible loss of vision has occurred.

Diffuse vascular leakage produces widespread macula oedema. If this persists microscopic fluid-filled cystic spaces may develop within the retina, a condition known as cystoid macula oedema. At the fovea these cystic spaces may coalesce producing partial thickness loss of retina tissue and a lamellar macula hole. Once this stage is reached vision is irretrievably impaired. Fluorescein angiography may sometimes be justified to search for an occult point of focal leakage or to establish the degree of coexistent ischaemia. A grid laser application over the area of retinal oedema is helpful in some patients.

PRE-PROLIFERATIVE RETINOPATHY

As retinal capillary non-perfusion becomes more widespread the fundal appearance grows more sinister. Haemorrhages tend to be larger, blotchy

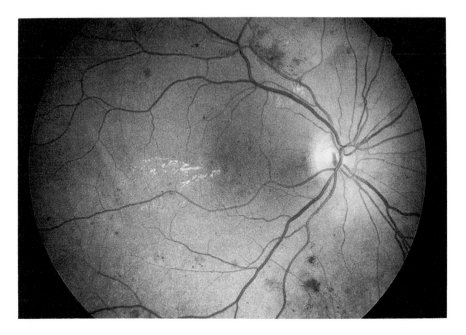

Figure 1.4. Exudative diabetic maculopathy of right eye. Vascular leakage temporal to the fovea is leading to the deposition of hard exudate within Henle's fibres, forming a spoke pattern. This is due to the peculiar anatomy of the retina at this site. Note also the different patterns of retinal haemorrhage. Flame-shaped or streaky haemorrhages lie within the nerve fibre layer, seen adjacent to the superotemporal vascular arcade. Dot haemorrhages lie deeper within the retinal structure

and more deeply seated within the retina. These may be associated with cotton wool spots which are present in larger numbers than in simple background retinopathy. The temporal macula region is particularly prone to ischaemia and often shows these features first. Between the haemorrhages the retina is pale and featureless. Intraretinal microvascular abnormalities (IRMAs) may be seen, particularly at the edge of areas of retinal capillary closure (Figure 1.2). These small vascular loops arise from capillaries or venules and represent either intraretinal shunt vessels or new vessel budding. Changes also appear in the larger vessels, particularly the retinal veins. These develop a variable calibre mimicking a string of sausages or beads. Venous loops are pathognomonic of pre-proliferative retinopathy and may be so extreme as almost to produce a vascular 'ox bow lake'.

Pre-proliferative retinopathy does not inevitably progress to proliferative retinopathy but the risk of this occurring may be as high as 50% within a year in some cases[6,7]. In view of this some ophthalmologists advocate laser treatment at this stage. Others would follow the patient up hawkishly and only treat should conversion to proliferative retinopathy occur. This approach spares those patients, who do not develop proliferative changes, the morbidity of laser treatment. However, if there is any doubt concerning the attendance of the patient at follow-up appointments then immediate treatment is certainly justified.

PROLIFERATIVE RETINOPATHY

If a sufficiently large proportion of the retinal capillary bed becomes non-perfused, thought to be of the order of at least 25%, then retinal neovascularization may occur. The precise mechanism for this is unknown. The most enduring theory suggests that the ischaemic retina produces diffusible blood vessel growth factors (vasoproliferative substances) in an attempt to rejuvenate retinal perfusion[8,9]. Unfortunately the new blood vessels so produced entirely fail to do this. Instead they tend to occur as fronds on the retinal surface, usually at the disc or adjacent to the major vascular arcades (Figures 1.5 and 1.6). The proliferation of these new vessels is particularly favoured when the vitreous remains in contact with the retina. The posterior surface of the vitreous then acts as a scaffold upon which the new vessels may grow and extend. If the vitreous has collapsed away from the retina (posterior vitreous detachment) before the new vessels appear, then they are unlikely to develop beyond vestigial vascular stumps.

New vessels lack the endothelial tight junctions characteristic of normal retinal vessels. This difference can be exploited by fluorescein angiography. If there is uncertainty as to the presence or location of retinal new vessels they may be identified by their tendency to leak fluorescein during angiography. This does not occur with normal vessels.

Unfortunately the development of proliferative retinopathy is usually asymptomatic and only becomes apparent when the fragile retinal new vessels bleed. All too often, therefore, it presents to the ophthalmologist at an advanced stage. If the initial bleeding is limited the patient may only notice a few 'floaters' but if extensive vitreal haemorrhage occurs there will be a sudden and precipitous fall in vision. Such vitreous haemorrhage is particularly likely if posterior vitreous detachment occurs in the presence of new vessels. The vessels are then rent as the posterior vitreous surface, into which they have become incorporated, moves forward.

Once vitreous haemorrhage is present it may be weeks or months before an adequate view of the fundus is regained and laser treatment can be given. In the meantime the retinopathy progresses unchecked increasing the risk of complications. A fibrous tissue web inevitably accompanies the

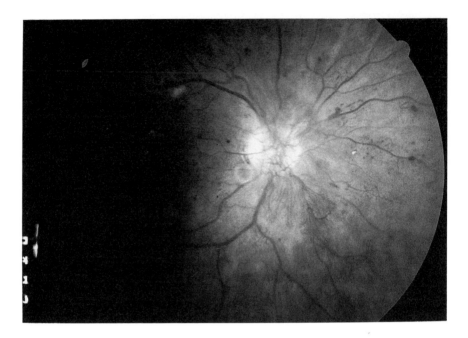

Figure 1.5. Proliferative diabetic retinopathy: new vessels at the disc (NVD). Fronds of fine wispy new vessels are seen extending from the right optic disc. (Courtesy of Professor D. McLeod and the Department of Clinical Imaging, Manchester Royal Eye Hospital)

proliferating new vessels and in time this undergoes contraction. The retina may then become puckered or tented up by tractional forces. In turn this may cause the retina to rip, converting a tractional retinal detachment into a more conventional rhegmatogenous detachment. These two types of detachment can be distinguished by the retinal contour. In a traction detachment the retina has a concave surface whereas in a rhegmatogenous detachment the retina is rippled and convex and relatively more mobile. At this stage the only hope for salvaging even a crude level of vision is vitreoretinal surgery.

SCREENING

For the screening of any disease to be worth while certain criteria need to be met[3,10]. This is particularly so in these days of limited health care resources[11]. These criteria include the following:

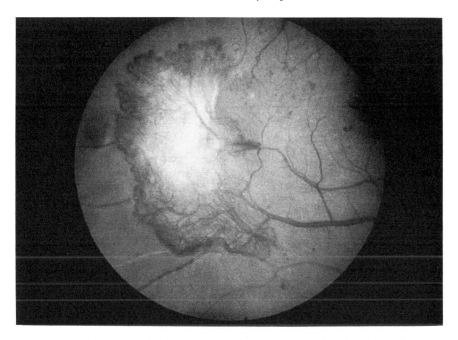

Figure 1.6. Proliferative diabetic retinopathy: new vessels elsewhere (NVE). A frond of new vessels is seen arising adjacent to a major vascular arcade in the retinal periphery. The reflectant whiteness is due to accompanying fibrous tissue proliferation. (Courtesy of Professor D. McLeod and the Department of Clinical Imaging, Manchester Royal Eye Hospital)

- The disorder for which screening is to be conducted should be well defined. That is, the nature of the disorder should be well understood and its clinical features easily identifiable.
- Estimates of the prevalence and rate of progression of the disorder should be known. This represents the size of the health problem and its threat within the population.

- The disorder should be asymptomatic, at least in its early stages, but if left untreated, lead to significant morbidity. This emphasizes the aim of screening, namely to detect the disorder early in its development so that treatment can be given to prevent progression and incapacity.

- An effective treatment for the condition should be available. It perhaps goes without saying that there is little point in detecting a disease, no matter how serious, if nothing can then be done about it.

- The screening method should be simple and safe.

- Screening should be able to discriminate between affected and un-affected individuals. That is, any screening programme should have a high sensitivity and specificity. It should be remembered, however, that screening is like a net trawling for fish. In practice some cases will always get through the net and be missed. Any attempt to catch every case (100% sensitivity) is likely to increase the catch of false positives (low specificity). In practice, therefore, the perfect screening programme probably does not exist.

- Finally, screening should be cost-effective. The resources needed to detect an individual with early treatable disease should be less than the resources that would be required to support and treat that patient once the disease had become manifest. In health care economic terms it is therefore usually more worth while to screen for relatively common conditions than for rare ones; unless the latter have particularly serious health implications if undetected.

When judged against these criteria diabetic retinopathy is eminently suitable for screening. It is relatively common and the more so the longer the duration of the diabetes. Both maculopathy and proliferative retino-pathy, the two blinding forms of diabetic retinopathy, may be present for some time before visual impairment occurs. This is particularly true of proliferative retinopathy where all may seem well until retinal new vessels bleed producing vitreous haemorrhage and a sudden and precipitous fall in vision. The unfavourable natural history of these conditions is well established from the pre-laser era. For example, bleeding new vessels at the disc if left untreated carry a 40% risk of severe visual loss within 2 years[10]. Detection and treatment of vision-threatening retinopathy at an early asymptomatic stage significantly improves the visual prognosis[13-16]. Indeed early treatment is vital. In the case of proliferative retinopathy, once vitreous haemorrhage has occurred laser treatment may be impos-sible for weeks or months. In the meantime the disease remains unchecked and further fibrovascular proliferation may occur. Repeated new vessel bleeding behind existing vitreous haemorrhage may prevent laser treat-ment altogether. The eye is then increasingly likely to suffer the complica-tions of vitreoretinal fibrosis and may require surgical intervention. The need for prompt treatment of exudative diabetic maculopathy is equally pressing. Focal vascular leakage is often very amenable to laser photo-coagulation with resolution of exudate and oedema. However, if exudate is allowed to accumulate at the fovea the retinal anatomy becomes perma-nently deranged with irreversible impairment of central vision.

Accepting that screening for diabetic retinopathy is worth while, how should it be done? In drawing up protocols for screening programmes two issues must be addressed. Firstly, which diabetic patients should be screened, and how often. Secondly, who should do the screening and with what tools?

The risk of developing diabetic retinopathy rises with the duration of the diabetes[3]. Retinopathy is rare in the first five years of the disease. In insulin-dependent diabetes (IDDM) the onset of the condition is usually well defined whereas this is often not the case with non-insulin-dependent diabetes (NIDDM). It is therefore recommended that all cases of NIDDM should have an annual fundus examination from time of diabetes diagnosis but that for those with IDDM this may be deferred until the diabetes has been present for 5 years.

Pregnancy is a particular risk factor for the development of diabetic retinopathy. If there is pre-existing mild retinopathy this may worsen abruptly and become vision threatening. A similar phenomenon may also occur in patients with longstanding poor diabetes control if this is suddenly corrected. In pregnancy good diabetes control is often more rigorously applied and these risk factors may compound. The ocular fundus should therefore be as much a part of the antenatal examinations as the uterine fundus. If retinopathy was documented before conception then examination by an ophthalmologist during the pregnancy is advisable[6,17,18].

The gold standard for detection of diabetic retinopathy is binocular stereoscopic slit lamp biomicroscopy conducted by an ophthalmologist through dilated pupils[3,16]. Unfortunately within the UK there are too few ophthalmologists, hard pressed with other ocular disorders, and too many diabetic patients for this to be a practical way of screening for retinopathy. Instead the role of the specialist must be to assess and treat those cases referred as a result of screening programmes conducted by other health-care professionals.

Potentially, screening may be conducted by general practitioners, diabetic physicians working in hospital clinics, optometrists, diabetic nurse practitioners or by retinal photography. Each brings particular advantages and disadvantages to the task.

SCREENING BY GENERAL PRACTITIONERS

Of all the health-care professionals potentially able to perform screening for retinopathy general practitioners (GPs) have the most direct and comprehensive contact with diabetic patients. They are in an ideal position to recruit and screen patients under their care. It should be a relatively easy matter to include an annual fundus examination in a patient's periodic general diabetic health check. However, the general practice working environment is often not ideal for ocular examination. In particular there is often too much ambient light and a lack of darkness. Diabetic mini clinics can help in this regard as they allow the surgery and working patterns to be adapted to the specific needs of diabetic assessment. Such clinics also have the advantage of concentrating pathology and sharpening clinical acumen. The ability to spot retinopathy and differentiate vision-threatening changes from trivia depends, in part, on reasonably frequent encounters with the disorder. This is a potential problem for GPs who may be responsible for a relatively small number of diabetic patients. Because of this some studies have found the ability of GPs to detect sight-threatening lesions to be as low as 10–20%[3]. However, performance can be dramatically improved by attendance at quite short courses of instruction including tuition in the use of the direct ophthalmoscopy[3]. Ultimately the effectiveness of screening by GPs depends very much on the motivation of individual practitioners.

SCREENING TECHNIQUE

The GP's main tools are the Snellen chart, the direct ophthalmoscope and the pinhole. With these the two most important observations to make are the best corrected visual acuity and the appearance of the optic disc. If the patient uses distance spectacles and these are not available, or if the acuity is less than 6/6, then it should be repeated with the patient looking through a pinhole. If the best visual acuity is 6/12 or less or has fallen by two lines or more since the last examination, diabetic maculopathy should be suspected. A fall in acuity of one line may merely reflect variation in test conditions. The optic disc is the commonest and most sinister site for the development of retinal new vessels in proliferative diabetic retinopathy.

These observations represent a minimum but are likely to detect most cases of immediately vision-threatening retinopathy. Ideally a full inspection of the ocular fundus should be made. This should be done through a dilated pupil, although in young patients with physiologically large pupils and clear ocular media this may not be necessary. The mydriatic of choice is Tropicamide (0.5% or 1%). This should produce adequate dilatation in 20 to 30 minutes lasting 3 to 4 hours. In darkly pigmented irides, and with the rigid irides of longstanding diabetes, 10% Phenylephrine may also be needed. Patients under 50 years of age should be warned about cycloplegia, loss of accommodation and the blurring of near vision caused by Tropicamide. There is also usually some blurring of distance vision in all patients due to an increase in ocular spherical aberration in the presence of a dilated pupil. In patients intending to drive following examination the visual acuity should be checked and, if less than 6/12, the patient should be advised not to drive until the pupil has returned to normal. It is good practice to warn patients of this possibility beforehand so that they may make appropriate arrangements.

In some elderly patients pupil dilatation caries the theoretical risk of inducing an acute angle closure glaucoma (AACG). This is most likely in eyes with hypermetropia ('longsightedness') and large cataractous lenses. A clue to the presence of hypermetropia is distance vision spectacle lenses that magnify. If the anterior chamber appears unduly shallow or the iris has a forward convexity then the patient should be dilated with caution. The latter feature can be tested by illuminating the eye from the side. If the iris is bowed forward it will cast a shadow on the side of the iris opposite the light. AACG is, however, a relatively rare occurrence. Overall the risk to vision from missing diabetic retinopathy is greater than the risk from glaucoma. If AACG does occur at least this is under medical supervision and referral to an ophthalmologist can be organized immediately.

Having dilated the pupil, examination of the ocular fundus should follow a logical sequence. Firstly, the disc is inspected looking for new vessels. The main superior and inferior temporal vascular arcades are then traced away from the disc. A similar scan is then made of the nasal vascular arcades. After the disc these vascular arcades are the next most common site for the development of new vessels. The macula, the area within the temporal arcades, is then inspected. Careful note should be made of the proximity of any retinopathy to the fovea. If within one disc diameter of the fovea this should be considered immediately vision threatening. If within two disc diameters of the fovea it should be considered potentially vision threatening. Finally, the peripheral retina is inspected.

SCREENING WITHIN HOSPITAL-BASED DIABETIC CLINICS

The screening tools needed in hospital diabetic clinics are the same as those used in general practice, namely the Snellen chart, the direct ophthalmoscope and the pinhole, and the same logic and techniques apply. Again retinal examination is facilitated by pupil dilatation and an adequately darkened environment. A hospital setting does, however, offer a number of advantages. The high throughput of diabetic patients means that medical staff who attend such clinics regularly will often encounter retinopathy and will be able to exercise their skills in its detection. This, combined with simple training programmes on direct ophthalmoscopy skills and retinopathy recognition, has been shown to improve the performance of consultant diabetologists from 50% detection of serious retinopathy to a level matching eye specialists[3]. It is also easier to develop liaison with the ophthalmologist from within a hospital.

A disadvantage of performing retinopathy screening in hospital clinics is that only a minority of diabetic patients attend them. Also multiple aspects of diabetes management are dealt with simultaneously. This, combined with a heavy workload, means that retinopathy may not receive specific consideration. A rapid turnover of junior medical staff may exacerbate this problem. Careful consideration must therefore be given to the organization of such clinics. Working practices should be adopted which facilitate efficient screening without compromising the smooth running of clinics. For example, nurses can record visual acuities and dilate pupils before patients see the doctor. Other options include involving ophthalmic clinical assistants, optometrists and fundus photography within these clinics.

SCREENING BY OPTOMETRISTS

At the time of writing patients with diabetes are entitled to free sight tests on the NHS, whenever clinically indicated. When dispensing with the universal free sight test in 1989 Parliament legislated this concession because it was recognized that optometrists had and could continue to provide a valuable role in the early detection of diabetic retinopathy. Indeed the terms under which optometrists conduct sight tests for the NHS oblige them to examine for and refer ocular pathology. The four-year training of optometrists therefore includes a substantial component on the techniques of fundal examination and recognition of abnormality. Once qualified an optometrist will examine ocular fundi day in, day out. The consequence of this is that the average optometrist is more confident and competent at detecting diabetic retinopathy and differentiating trivial from vision-threatening changes than is the average general practitioner or non-ophthalmologist. Because of the lamentable ophthalmic training in most UK medical schools this is particularly true of those GPs who have not spent time in an ophthalmology post after graduation. Crucially, screening for diabetic retinopathy by optometrists has been shown to be reliable[3,19].

Optometrists have the further advantages that their working environment is specifically designed for ocular examination and they have no requirement to check any other aspect of the diabetes. They are permitted by law to use dilating drops. For many patients a visit to the optometrist is also more convenient and less threatening than a visit to the doctor or the hospital. An annual visit to the optometrist is therefore a simple, available, cheap and effective way of screening for diabetic retinopathy and should be encouraged.

There is particular value in developing good relations and close liaison locally between optometrists and GPs. The latter ought not to be timid or overly proud of tapping into the skills of their non-medical colleagues. Potentially the optometrist's involvement in ocular assessment may be organized in a number of ways, although the GP must always remain in overall charge of patient care. The optometrist might take part in a diabetic mini clinic within GP health centres, as do chiropodists. Alternatively, individual patients might be sent by their GP to an optometrist for a fundal report. More formal optometrist-based screening schemes have been tried in some areas. Precise arrangements and protocols must be tailored to local circumstances and acceptable to all involved. Such a scheme might operate, for example, by requiring optometrists to report on the fundal findings of every diabetic patient examined. Specially designed report forms indicating specific diagnostic criteria make this task simple and uniform. Completed reports could then be forwarded to a screening coordinator for vetting by an ophthalmologist, with a copy to the GP for his/her information. A scheme like this has the advantage of involving the expertise of an ophthalmologist enabling him/her to advise the GP on those cases likely to require referral for specialist clinical examination. Feedback to the screening optometrist can be provided and the channels of communication between optometrist, GP and specialist are kept well oiled.

The optometrists' reports can also be used to build up an epidemiological picture of retinopathy in the local diabetic population. Such schemes do though need careful planning including training and discussion sessions with local optometrists and GPs.

SCREENING BY RETINAL PHOTOGRAPHY

The ocular fundus may be assessed using photographs as well as by direct visualization. The best photographic images are obtained using multiple stereoscopic views taken over a wide area of the fundus on high-quality 35 mm slide film. This technique is used when conducting research into diabetic retinopathy but it is too complex and time consuming to be a practical method for screening. For this, non-mydriatic fundus photography is more appropriate. The non-mydriatic camera produces either a colour Polaroid print or transparency of the central 45 degrees of the fundus[3,20]. This view includes the optic disc, the major vascular arcades and the macula, i.e. that part of the fundus where vision-threatening retinopathy is most likely to occur. As its name suggests, photographs are usually obtained without dilating the pupil. Instead of the bright visible viewing light used in a standard fundus camera the non-mydriatic camera has a built-in infrared-sensitive video. A small TV screen allows the operator to align and focus the retinal view without inducing pupil constriction. The photograph itself is taken using a conventional flash. Photographs of an acceptable quality can be obtained from up to 90% of eyes[21]. Poorer quality photographs tend to occur in older patients, and this is probably related to the development of cataract and the reduction in pupil size that occurs with ageing[21]. In this situation a better photograph may be obtained after dilating the pupil. The description of the camera as 'non-mydriatic' in no way bars the use of dilating drops where appropriate.

In a large study comprising non-mydriatic Polaroid retinal photography with non-ophthalmologists working in hospital diabetic clinics the camera was found to be at least as good as direct ophthalmoscopy, performed through dilated pupils, in detecting retinal new vessels and better in detecting exudative maculopathy[22].

The non-mydriatic camera can also be used to assist screening in both general practice and hospital diabetic clinics. For general practice, particularly those serving rural communities, the camera can be housed in a mobile screening unit[23]. Running costs can then be shared and the camera put to best and most efficient use. However, optimal photographic results are likely to be obtained by establishing the camera at a fixed site. It can then be accommodated within a purpose-built and controlled environment and run by a designated team familiar with its operation. This may be within a hospital diabetic clinic or a diabetes care centre.

Retinal photography has further advantages. Although the pictures are taken by technicians or nurse practitioners, the expertise of an ophthalmologist can be employed in their interpretation. The ability to avoid the use of dilating drops in most cases makes it a convenient and acceptable screening method for patients. The photographs also provide a permanent record of the state of retinopathy and can be used as a teaching aid.

The non-mydriatic camera does though have a number of potential disadvantages. There are costs involved in purchasing and running the instrument as well as employing staff to operate it. However, a study in the USA has shown that primary care screening using 45 degree retinal photography was a more cost-effective means of screening than using ophthalmologists, physicians or nurse practitioners, especially if the photographs were taken through dilated pupils[24].

Despite pupil dilation, good quality photographs cannot be obtained in a minority of patients. If fine new vessels are raised above the retinal surface they will be out of focus and are liable to be missed. Also vision-threatening retinopathy outside the 45 degree field will not be seen. However, in both these situations there are usually other visible features of gross retinal ischaemia that would raise suspicion of a high risk of retinal neovascularization.

MANAGEMENT AND THERAPY

The management of diabetic retinopathy falls into three phases: prevention, screening and treatment. Screening has been dealt with in the preceding section. Efforts to prevent retinopathy can be directed either at controlling the diabetes itself or the microvascular abnormalities it produces. One might logically expect that mimicking physiological insulin profiles in diabetic patients and reducing blood glucose levels to normal would prevent retinopathy and the other complications of diabetes. Demonstrating whether or not this is the case in practice has been difficult because of the long-term follow-up required. Several studies have suggested that good control of diabetes in the early years after diagnosis does discourage the development of retinopathy but that abruptly tightening control tends to worsen retinopathy, at least in the short term[6,16,25,26]. The issue has now probably been settled by the 'Diabetes Control and Complications Trial' (DCCT)[27]. This study followed nearly 1500 patients over a mean of 6.5 years. In those patients with no retinopathy at the start of the study intensive therapy (at least thrice daily insulin) reduced the onset of retinopathy by 76% when compared with similar patients receiving only once or twice daily insulin. For patients with mild retinopathy at the outset, progression of retinopathy was slowed by 54% when using the intensive insulin regime as compared to those using a conventional regime. The key parameter appears to be the level of glycosylated haemoglobin, which reflects the true level of hyperglycaemia control. This should be kept within or close to the normal range. The downside of such tight diabetes control is an increase in the incidence of hypoglycaemic episodes. The results of this study should, however, be applied with caution to patients with established retinopathy or chronically poor diabetes control. It bears repetition that suddenly 'improving' control in such patients may dangerously worsen their retinopathy and should therefore be avoided.

In addition to hyperglycaemia, attention should also be given to the other risk factors known to potentiate diabetic retinopathy[6]. The most important of these is strict control of systemic hypertension. As discussed previously, pregnancy may induce proliferative retinopathy and the prospective mother should be counselled about this.

Attempts have been made to develop a pharmacological agent capable of preventing the characteristic microvascular abnormalities of diabetic retinopathy. This research has largely been based on animal models and Aldose Reductase Inhibitors (ARI)[28]. Aldose reductase is the enzyme responsible for the conversion, via the Polyol pathway, of sugars such as glucose and galactose to their respective sugar alcohols, sorbitol and galactitol. Dogs and rats fed galactose-rich diets develop vascular endothelial thickening identical to that found in human diabetics. These histopathological changes can be inhibited if the animals are also given ARI. Unfortunately, trials in humans have so far been disappointing. Two possible reasons for this are that the distribution of aldose reductase is different in man from that in dogs and rats, or the available ARI, at the doses used, failed to get into the eye in sufficient amounts[28].

Theoretically, proliferative retinopathy might be inhibited by the intra-vitreal injection of inhibitory vascular growth factors. Also the induction of posterior vitreous detachment prior to the appearance of retinal new vessels would remove the scaffold upon which they proliferate. However, neither of these therapeutic approaches is currently feasible.

The mainstay of current treatment for diabetic retinopathy is retinal photocoagulation. Initial trials in the late 1970s used intense non-coherent white light from a xenon arc[13,14,16]. This had the disadvantage of produ-cing large full thickness retinal burns which made macula treatment parti-cularly hazardous. Today photocoagulation is achieved using coherent laser light. There are a variety of lasers available but the most widely used in the UK remains the argon green laser (wavelength 514 nm). The laser light can be delivered to the retina through a contact lens with the patient sitting at a slit lamp, through an indirect ophthalmoscope or from within the eye during vitreoretinal surgery (Figures 1.7 and 1.8).

Exudative maculopathy and proliferative retinopathy are the two prin-cipal treatable forms of diabetic retinopathy but they require quite differ-ent types of laser treatment. In exudative maculopathy the aim is to seal the sites of vascular leakage threatening the fovea. These sites are often

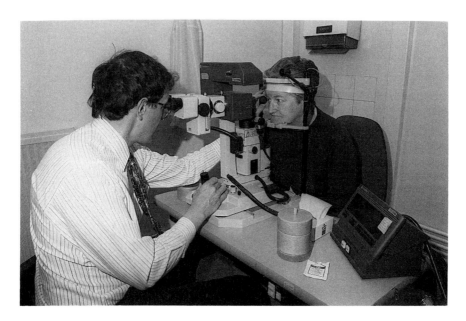

Figure 1.7. The application of retinal laser photocoagulation using a slit lamp and contact lens delivery system. (Courtesy of the Department of Clinical Imaging, Manchester Royal Eye Hospital)

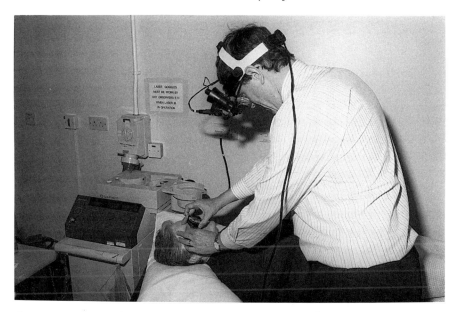

Figure 1.8. The application of retinal laser photocoagulation using the indirect ophthalmoscope. (Courtesy of the Department of Clinical Imaging, Manchester Royal Eye Hospital)

identified by rings of yellowy exudate (circinates). Focal laser burns are applied to the points of leakage, for example the centre of a circinate exudate. Because of the proximity of the fovea accuracy in delivery of the laser is vital and the treatment is best performed at the slit lamp. The viewing contact lens assists in stabilizing the eye, a high degree of magnification can be obtained and the size of individual retinal burns is easily controlled. Within the macula, burns of 50 to 200 microns (μm) diameter are used, with the smaller size being applied nearer the fovea. A typical treatment is unlikely to exceed 100 burns. Laser power, measured in milliwatts, depends on the clarity of the ocular media, the idiosyncrasies of the machine, presence of retinal oedema and haemorrhage and the size of burn. If local vascular leakage is successfully stemmed adjacent retinal exudate will resorb over the course of a few months.

Diffuse vascular leakage leading to widespread macula oedema is more difficult to treat. However, in some patients the application of very gently low-power laser burns in a grid pattern over the area of oedema can be helpful. In the absence of vascular leakage, laser can do nothing for macula ischaemia.

The aim of treatment in proliferative retinopathy is to induce regression

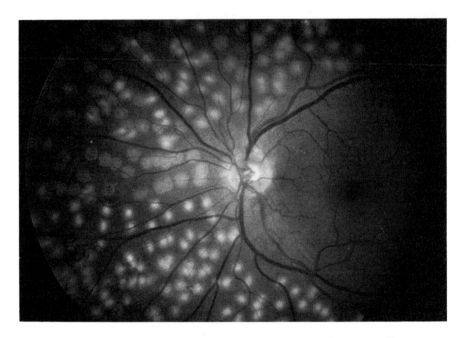

Figure 1.9. Panretinal laser photocoagulation (PRP). Fresh non-confluent argon laser burns are shown, scattered throughout the retina but sparing the macula

of retinal new vessels. This may require several thousands of laser burns. These burns are not applied to the new vessels themselves but rather to their cause, the ischaemic peripheral retina. This widespread peripheral retinal laser ablation is known as 'Panretinal Photocoagulation' or PRP (Figure 1.9). The macula is left untreated to preserve central vision.

Laser energy is principally absorbed by the melanin pigment of the retinal pigment epithelium and choroid. These structures lie beneath the neurosensory retina. As a burn develops the overlying photoreceptors and outer retina layers are destroyed. Full thickness and confluent retinal burns should be avoided so as to preserve the nerve fibre layer on the innermost surface of the retina. If the nerve fibre layer is damaged then vision will be lost, not only from the site of the laser burn itself, but also from a small wedge of the visual field conveyed by the affected nerve fibre bundle. Nevertheless, even a perfectly applied PRP is likely to cause some constriction of the visual field or reduction in peripheral visual sensitivity, and patients should be warned of this. Extensive treatment to both eyes may disqualify the patient from driving. (The DVLC currently require a combined visual field of 120 degrees horizontally and 20 degrees above and below fixation.) Laser treatment may also impair dark adaptation and colour sensitivity. The morbidity of treatment, however, should be seen in the context of the high risk of blindness without treatment.

The mechanism by which PRP causes regression of retinal new vessels is uncertain. The simplistic explanation is that ischaemic retina liberates some vasoproliferative substance. By destroying this ischaemic retina the production of vasoproliferative substances is halted and the stimulus to new vessel growth is removed. As an alternative some have proposed that destruction of the outer retinal layers causes retinal thinning. The metabolism of the remaining retina can then be supported by diffusion from the choroid thus relieving retinal ischaemia. The current hypothesis, however, suggests that laser treatment alters the balance of substances influencing blood vessel growth. This may be by stimulating the retinal pigment epithelium to produce vasoinhibitory factors.

Despite aggressive laser treatment progressive loss of vision in some eyes cannot be halted. Formerly this would have resulted in certain blindness but since the advent of vitreoretinal surgery vision in these eyes can now sometimes be salvaged. Persisting vitreous haemorrhage is relatively easily dealt with by vitrectomy. Once a clear view of the ocular fundus has been restored laser treatment can be given. This may be performed from within the eye at the time of vitrectomy (endolaser).

The growth of retinal new vessels is usually accompanied by a proliferation of fibrous tissue. Even if the vessels regress fibrous bands will persist. Over time these tend to contract producing tractional retinal detachments. The retinal distortion so produced may itself impair vision, however retinal tears may also develop leading to a rhegmatogenous retinal detachment. Surgical intervention is then the only means of redeeming the situation. More subtle fibrosis may develop over the macula in the form of an epiretinal membrane. This also tends to contract producing puckering of the macula and distortion of central vision. If this is particularly troublesome surgical peeling of the membrane may be justified. Unfortunately surgery has nothing to offer end stage diabetic maculopathy.

With profound retinal ischaemia, particularly in association with a persisting retinal detachment, new vessels may proliferate on the iris (rubeosis iridis) and in the anterior chamber angle. The latter causes obstruction to aqueous drainage and the intraocular pressure rises to a high level; a condition known as 'rubeotic glaucoma'. Such an eye may become painful as well as blind. Ocular comfort is the only objective of treatment in this situation. This can often be achieved with topical steroid and atropine. Unfortunately, however, some eyes do eventually require enucleation.

Screening, the wider availability of laser technology and improvements in surgical techniques offer the potential for progressively reducing the proportion of diabetics that become blind. However, the increasing prevalence of diabetes makes this an ever increasing challenge.

OTHER OCULAR COMPLICATIONS OF DIABETES

In addition to retinopathy, diabetes may cause a variety of other problems to the eye and the visual system. Many of these are related to disease of blood vessels which is so much a feature of diabetes. They include a higher incidence of retinal artery and venous occlusion, infarction of the optic disc (anterior ischaemic optic neuropathy), extraocular nerve palsies and cerebrovascular accidents affecting the brain stem eye movement coordination centres and the visual cortex. The disturbance to carbohydrate metabolism also impinges on the integrity of the crystalline lens of the eye. Fluctuations in serum glucose levels and the associated osmotic effects on the lens can cause significant changes in refractive error from day to day. Nuclear sclerotic cataract tends to occur at an earlier age in diabetic patients though true acute onset cortical 'diabetic cataract' is a rare phenomenon.

REFERENCES

1 Department of Health and Social Security. Blindness and partial sight in England 1969–76. London: HMSO, 1979. (Reports on Public Health and Medical Subjects, No. 129.)
2 Ghafour IM, Allan D, Foulds WS. Common causes of blindness and visual handicap in the west of Scotland. *Br J Ophthalmol* 1983; **67**: 209–13.
3 MacCuish AC. Early detection and screening for diabetic retinopathy. *Eye* 1993; 7: 254–9.
4 Barnett AH. Origins of the microangiopathic changes in diabetes. *Eye* 1993; **7**: 218–22.
5 Garner A. Histopathology of diabetic retinopathy in man. *Eye* 1993; 7: 250–3.
6 Ulbig MRW, Hamilton AMP. Factors influencing the natural history of diabetic retinopathy. *Eye* 1993; 7: 242–9.
7 Miller SM (Ed.). *Clinical Ophthalmology*. London: Wright, 1987. Kohner E, Hamilton AMP. Vascular retinopathies: the management of diabetic retinopathy: 238–43.
8 Cotlier E, Weinreb R. Growth factors in retinal diseases: proliferative vitreoretinopathy, proliferative diabetic retinopathy, and retinal degeneration. *Survey Ophthalmol* 1992; **36**: 373–84.
9 Forrester JV, Shafiee A, Schroder S, Knott R, McIntosh L. The role of growth factors in proliferative diabetic retinopathy. *Eye* 1993; 7: 276–87.
10 Rohan TE, Frost CD, Wald NJ. Prevention of blindness by screening for diabetic retinopathy: a quantitative assessment. *BMJ* 1989; **299**: 1198–201.
11 Calman KC. Screening policy in the NHS. Department of Health Chief Medical Officer's update No. 2, May 1994: 4.

12 The Diabetic Retinopathy Study Research Group. Four risk factors for severe visual loss in diabetic retinopathy. *Arch Ophthalmol* 1979; **97**: 654–5.

13 British Multicentre Study Group. Photocoagulation for proliferative diabetic retinopathy: a randomised controlled clinical trial using the xenon arc. *Diabetologia* 1984; **26**: 109–15.

14 British Multicentre Study Group. Photocoagulation for diabetic maculopathy: a randomised controlled clinical trial using the xenon arc. *Diabetes* 1983; **32**: 1010–16.

15 Flanagan DW. Current management of established diabetic eye disease. *Eye* 1993; **7**: 302–8.

16 Kohner EM. Diabetic retinopathy (fortnightly review). *BMJ* 1993; **307**: 1195–9.

17 Jovanovic-Peterson L, Peterson CM. Diabetic retinopathy. *Clin Obstet Gynecol* 1991; **34**: 516–25.

18 Phelps RL, Sakol P, Metzger BE, Jampol LM, Freinkel N. Changes in diabetic retinopathy during pregnancy. *Arch Ophthalmol* 1986; **104**: 1806–10.

19 Burns-Cox CJ, Dean Hart JC. Screening of diabetics for retinopathy by ophthalmic opticians. *BMJ* 1985; **290**: 1052–4.

20 Ryder RE, Vora JP, Atiea JA, Owens DR, Hayes TM, Young S. Possible new method to improve detection of diabetic retinopathy: Polaroid non-mydriatic retinal photography. *BMJ* 1985; 1256–7.

21 Heaven CJ, Cansfield J, Shaw KM. The quality of photographs produced by the non-mydriatic fundus camera in a screening programme for diabetic retinopathy: a 1 year prospective study. *Eye* 1993; **7**: 787–90.

22 Taylor R, Lovelock L, Tunbridge WMG, Alberti KGMM, Brackenridge RG, Stephenson P, Young E. Comparison of non-mydriatic retinal photography with ophthalmoscopy in 2159 patients: mobile retinal camera study. *BMJ* 1990; **301**: 1243–7.

23 Leese GP, Newton RW, Jung RT, Haining W, Ellingford A. Screening for diabetic retinopathy in a widely spaced population using non-mydriatic fundus photography in a mobile unit. *Diabetic Medicine* 1992; **9**: 459–62.

24 Lairson DR, Pugh JA, Kapadia AS, Lorimor RJ, Jacobson J, Velez R. Cost effectiveness of alternative methods for diabetic retinopathy screening. *Diabetes Care* (United States) 1992; **15**: 1369–77.

25 Brinchmann-Hansen O, Dahl-Jorgensen K, Sandvik L, Hanssen KF. Blood glucose concentrations and progression of diabetic retinopathy: the seven year results of the Oslo study. *BMJ* 1992; **304**: 19–22.

26 Kohner EM. The effect of diabetic control on diabetic retinopathy. *Eye* 1993; **7**: 309–11.

27 The Diabetes Control and Complications Trial Research Group. The effect of intensive treatment of diabetes on the development and progression of long-term complications in insulin-dependent diabetes mellitus. *N Engl J Med* 1993; **329**: 977–86.

28 Lightman S. Does aldose reductase have a role in the development of the ocular complications of diabetes? *Eye* 1993; **7**: 238–41.

2

Diabetic Renal Disease

G. F. WATTS

University Department of Medicine,
Royal Perth Hospital, Western Australia

INTRODUCTION

While the introduction of insulin therapy in 1924 improved the immediate outlook of thousands of patients with diabetes mellitus, it subsequently uncovered the ogre of the long-term complications of the disease[1]. Prospective studies in diabetic clinics on both sides of the Atlantic subsequently demonstrated the high incidence rate of occlusive vascular disease, retinopathy, neuropathy and nephropathy. These are now collectively recognized to be due to a specific degenerative lesion of blood vessels referred to as diabetic angiopathy. That renal involvement occurred in diabetes mellitus was recognized quite early on by nineteenth-century physicians, most notably by Cotunnius and by Bright. Renal disease is particularly important in diabetic patients because it provides the nexus for expression of other long-term complications. This chapter will describe the problem posed by overt diabetic nephropathy and will then focus on its prevention through the detection and treatment of microalbuminuria.

RENAL STRUCTURE AND FUNCTION

The kidney is a vital organ that fulfils several important functions including the control of water and electrolyte metabolism, the regulation of arterial blood pressure, and the excretion of both endogenously produced

Diabetic Complications. Edited by K. M. Shaw
© 1996 John Wiley & Sons Ltd

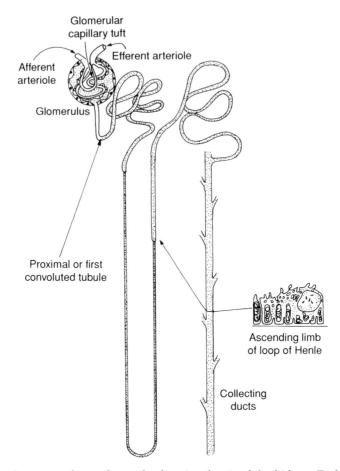

Figure 2.1. Structure of a nephron, the functional unit of the kidney. Diabetic renal disease primarily affects the glomerulus

and exogenously ingested toxic chemicals. Its functional unit is the nephron of which there are approximately 750 000 in each kidney, the numbers declining with age. The nephron is comprised of a glomerulus and renal tubular system (Figure 2.1). The glomerulus consists of a bunch of capillaries which receive blood from the afferent arteriole (derived from the renal artery) and are drained by the efferent arteriole. The wall of the glomerulus is effectively a filtration barrier which under pressure separates blood cells and large molecules from small molecules and water. The latter form the so-called glomerular ultrafiltrate. The rate at which this is formed is a measure of renal function and is referred to as the glomerular

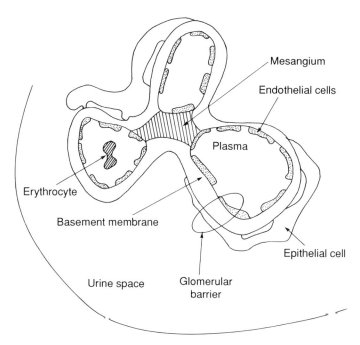

Figure 2.2. Diagrammatic high powered cross-sectional representation of the glomerular capillary lobule of kidney. To get into the urine space albumin has to pass from the plasma across the endothelial cells, basement membrane and epithelial cells. In diabetic renal disease the basement membrane increases in thickness and the mesangium expands to invade the glomerular barrier. Increase in albumin in the urine reflects damage to the glomerular barrier

filtration rate (GFR); normal GFR ranges between 80 and 120 ml/min. Figure 2.2 shows in cross-section the structure of the glomerular capillary lobule of the kidney: the glomerular capillary barrier essentially consists of the inner lining of endothelial cells, the basement membrane and the outer layer of the epithelial cells; the supporting tissue or mesangium is not part of the barrier normally, but encroaches on it in diabetic glomerular disease. Pathological changes in the structure and function of the filtration barrier are reflected by changes in the chemical constituents of the glomerular ultrafiltrate, one of the most clinically important of which, in the context of this chapter, is albumin. With an intact glomerular capillary wall, the size and shape of the albumin molecule restricts its passage into the ultrafiltrate and the urine. Measurement of albumin excretion provides a useful index of the integrity of the glomerular barrier or the extent of its 'leakiness'. The renal tubular system modifies the glomerular ultrafiltrate by controlling water reabsorption in the proximal convoluted tubule, the loop of Henle, distal convoluted tubule and the collecting ducts. Given that regulation of water excretion involves other parts of the nephron, measurement of urinary albumin excretion rate is a better reflector of the integrity of the filtration barrier, and hence glomerular function, than measurement of urinary albumin concentration alone.

OVERT DIABETIC NEPHROPATHY

CLINICAL DIAGNOSIS

The cardinal sign of overt diabetic nephropathy is persistent proteinuria[2] in excess of 0.5 g/24 h. This is referred to as macroproteinuria, or clinical proteinuria, and is classically detectable by indicator dye-binding methods such as Albustix; a positive Albustix Dipstix test is equivalent to a concentration of urinary protein (chiefly albumin) of 300 mg/l. The syndrome of overt nephropathy in insulin-dependent patients also invariably includes systemic hypertension, retinopathy, neuropathy, macrovascular disease and elevated serum creatinine concentration.

HISTOPATHOLOGICAL FEATURES

Typically, the microscopic features that the pathologist notes are thickening of the glomerular basement membrane, expansion of the mesangium (the supporting tissue of the glomerulus) and fibrotic changes in the afferent and efferent arterioles. These lesions may be restricted to a specific area or be diffusely scattered throughout the glomerulus, being referred to as nodular and diffuse glomerular sclerosis, respectively.

NATURAL HISTORY

Diabetic patients who develop persistent proteinuria have a high mortality due to both uraemia and cardiovascular disease[3]. Intermittent proteinuria heralds persistent proteinuria by up to several years[2]. The latter is followed by progressive loss of renal function manifest as a steady increase in urinary protein loss and an unremitting decline in GFR. Once serum creatinine concentration reaches 200 μmol, the GFR falls at a mean rate of 1 ml/min/month with acceleration of other long-term diabetic complications. The major determinant for the fall in GFR and rise in proteinuria is blood pressure, there still being much debate concerning the relative roles of dietary protein and glycaemic control. By the time end-stage-renal-failure (ESRF) is reached, typically 7 years after the onset of persistent proteinuria, insulin-dependent patients are aged less than 50 years with duration of diabetes between 20 and 25 years. Clinically they have advanced proliferative retinopathy, severe peripheral neuropathy and widespread macrovascular disease. The natural history in non-insulin-dependent patients is probably similar to insulin-dependent diabetics, but a greater proportion of the former die from cardiovascular disease before reaching ESRF.

EPIDEMIOLOGY: SIZE OF THE PROBLEM

The prevalence of clinical proteinuria in diabetic patients ranges between 4.4 and 33%. In insulin-dependent diabetics it increases with time, with the highest incidence (*c.* 3%/year) being found between those with 16–20 years' duration of diabetes. Up to 70% of insulin-dependent diabetic patients, however, never develop overt diabetic nephropathy, for reasons which are unknown. The cumulative risk in non-insulin-dependent diabetic patients varies with ethnic group and in the UK is highest among those of Asian origin. In the UK it is also estimated that approximately 600 young insulin-dependent diabetic patients develop renal failure each year, and these account for 15% of all deaths in diabetics aged less than 50 years[3]. Studies from Denmark show that the relative mortality in insulin-dependent diabetic patients aged 20–40 years with persistent proteinuria is 25- to 100-fold greater than in patients without proteinuria, and that a significant proportion of the excess is due to macrovascular disease. In the USA the percentage of all new cases accepted for ESRF treatment due to diabetic nephropathy increased from 7% in 1974 to 25% in 1980. By contrast, in the UK it only increased from 1.5% to 11.1% over the same period. There is evidently still a shortfall of diabetic patients receiving treatment for ESRF in the UK[3]. This is a policy decision that is economically led and probably reflects the specifically high morbidity and mortality of diabetics receiving ESRF treatment. In the USA the annual costs of treatment and care in diabetic patients in 1989 were estimated at $200 billion.

THERAPY

Several therapies may be employed to retard the increase in proteinuria and fall in GFR in diabetics with overt nephropathy[4]. Of these the most important is control of elevated arterial blood pressure. The diagnosis and treatment of hypertension is essential and the most promising drugs appear to be the angiotensing-converting enzyme inhibitors. Clear benefit from very tight glycaemic control and low protein diets has not been established. Once a diabetic patient enters ESRF the two options are renal dialysis or renal transplantation (preferably from a living related donor). Despite recent advances, the outcome of renal replacement therapy in diabetic patients remains worse than in non-diabetics. This is again related to the associated vascular, neuropathic and infective co-complications.

CONCLUSION

Diabetic nephropathy is a serious and common long-term complication of diabetes mellitus. It threatens the health and life of up to half of patients who develop insulin-dependent diabetes in youth and a smaller but significant number of those with non-insulin-dependent diabetes. Available medical therapy has little impact on the decline of established nephropathy to ESRF. The management of patients is severely hampered by coexistent atherosclerosis, retinopathy and neuropathy. The financial costs imposed by treatment and care are immense. There is clearly a major demand to identify and treat patients at the earliest possible stage of renal involvement. This provides a powerful rationale and impetus for establishing preventive programmes involving the screening, monitoring and treatment of patients with very early diabetic nephropathy.

DIABETIC RENAL DISEASE: A MULTISTAGE DISORDER

The development of established diabetic nephropathy and ESRF is preceded by several changes in kidney structure and function which take place over a period of several years[2,4]. The initial abnormalities involved are an increase in kidney size and function, referred to as glomerular hypertrophy and hyperfunction, respectively. Almost all patients then develop glomerular basement membrane thickening and expansion of the mesangium. In this second stage urinary albumin excretion is normal, but mild elevation may be unmasked by moderate physical exercise and poor glycaemic control. A proportion of patients then develop persistently elevated urinary albumin excretion (microalbuminuria) which heralds the progression to clinically overt renal disease, typically 15 to 20 years after the onset of diabetes in insulin-dependent patients. If hypertension and poor metabolic control are not treated these patients will proceed to the subsequent stage of overt nephropathy, characterized by clinical proteinuria, hypertension and reduction in GFR together with advanced glomerular lesions. After a period of a few years the patient then enters the final stage of generalized glomerular shutdown and ESRF when the GFR is <10 ml/min and renal replacement therapy is required for survival. At all stages of the foregoing spectrum it is important to realize that any type of renal disease (e.g. pyelonephritis, renal calculi) may affect the diabetic patient in the same way as the non-diabetic.

EARLY RENAL CHANGES IN THE DIABETIC KIDNEY

Several early renal abnormalities[4] have been described and these are summarized in Table 2.1.

GLOMERULAR FILTRATION RATE AND RENAL BLOOD FLOW

The GFR is well known to be moderately increased in most insulin-dependent patients. The reason for this is unknown but may be due to alterations in renal blood flow, renal structure and blood glucose control. Both short- and long-term correction of hyperglycaemia is known to significantly lower both renal blood flow and GFR. Several workers have proposed that increase in renal blood flow and GFR (referred to as hyperfiltration) may determine the onset and progression of diabetic glomerular disease. The hyperfiltration hypothesis, however, needs to be reconciled with the finding that all long-term, insulin-dependent patients have elevated GFR and some glomerular structural changes, but only approximately 30% develop clinically significant nephropathy. However, there is evidence that in patients with microalbuminuria persistent hyperfiltration accelerates the deterioration in renal function.

RENAL STRUCTURE

Two types of early structural changes are seen in the diabetic kidney. The first are changes in the fine structure, so-called ultrastructural changes, and the second are changes in the gross structure of the kidney.

Table 2.1. Some of the early renal changes in diabetes mellitus

---

- ↑ Albumin excretion
- ↑ Glomerular filtration rate
- ↑ Renal blood flow
- ↑ Filtration fraction
- ↑ Renal size
- ↑ Glomerular basement membrane (GBM)
- ↑ Mesangial expansion
- ↓ GBM anionic charge

Ultrastructural Changes

The ultrastructural hallmark of early diabetic glomerular disease is thickening of the basement membrane and proliferation of the mesangial tissue. These changes may be reversible by improved glycaemic control, as shown in both human and animal experiments. The significance of altered glomerular ultrastructure, however, remains open to question, since advanced changes can occur in many diabetic patients who never develop overt nephropathy. It is, therefore, not surprising that an association between ultrastructural changes and microalbuminuria has not been consistently demonstrated.

Gross Structural Changes

Standard imaging techniques show that whole kidney size is increased in diabetic patients. This is due to increase in the size of both the glomeruli and renal tubules. The mechanism for increase in renal size is unknown but may be due to the effects of glucose or growth promoting factors, such as insulin and growth hormone. Strict metabolic control improves gross structural abnormality.

GLOMERULAR BARRIER BIOCHEMISTRY

The glomerulus restricts the passage of plasma proteins into the urinary space, owing to the negative charge and restricted pore size of the filtration barrier. In early diabetic renal disease there is a marked reduction in the negative charge of the glomerular barrier. In consequence, negatively charged large molecules accumulate within the membrane and cause glomerular damage. Recent research suggests that poor glycaemic control and genetic factors reduce the metabolism of a complex biochemical molecule called heparan sulphate proteoglycan, and that this reduces the charge of the membrane and leads to early diabetic nephropathy. This interesting concept needs to be further researched.

MICROPROTEINURIA

Several research workers detected early on an elevated excretion of plasma proteins in the urine of diabetic patients[2]. Developments in sophisticated and sensitive analytical methods allowed very small quantities of plasma proteins to be detected in the urine, referred to collectively as microproteinuria. The major plasma protein in the urine is albumin, but small amounts of other proteins such as immunoglobulins may also be detected. The pattern of urinary protein excretion in diabetes mellitus suggests that the damage is almost exclusively glomerular and not tubular. Microproteinuria in diabetes, therefore, reflects an elevated urinary excretion of a wide variety of plasma proteins, predominant among which is albumin. For sometime this was not considered to be of clinical significance, but there is now good evidence that it is a powerful predictor of overt nephropathy and cardiovascular mortality in both insulin-dependent and non-insulin-dependent patients[5-7].

MICROALBUMINURIA

HISTORICAL BACKGROUND

In the early 1960s Professor Harry Keen's Group at Guy's Hospital developed a technique called radio-immunoassay for measuring very low concentrations of albumin in urine which they termed microalbuminuria, or subclinical albuminuria, in an epidemiological survey in Bedford. Newly diagnosed non-insulin-dependent patients were found to have higher urinary albumin excretion than non-diabetics and a link was reported with poor glycaemic control and high blood pressure. Interest in microalbuminuria picked up a decade or so later and extensive work was carried out in the UK and in Denmark in insulin-dependent patients. A significant early finding was that improvement in glycaemic control with insulin could reverse microalbuminuria, but the modest elevations in albumin excretion were not considered to be of major clinical importance until 1982. It was then that Viberti and colleagues and Parving and colleagues independently published prospective evidence showing that microalbuminuria was a powerful predictor of future overt nephropathy in insulin-dependent patients[24]. These two seminal results spawned the vast body of research now aimed at the detection and prevention of diabetic renal disease.

DEFINITION

Microalbuminuria is a level of urinary albumin excretion in excess of the upper limit of the reference range for non-diabetic subjects and which is classically undetectable by the Albustix Dipstix test[2]. Urinary albumin concentration should be measured by an immunochemical method with a lower limit of detection of at least 3 mg/l, Albustix showing a positive result at around 250–350 mg/l. Albumin excretion should be expressed as an excretion rate (μg/min or mg/24h) or as an albumin/creatinine ratio (mg/mmol) in preference to a concentration (mg/l), since the latter is affected not only by glomerular leakiness but also by the control of water metabolism by the kidney[8]. Reference ranges in non-diabetic subjects for urinary albumin excretion depend on several factors of which the most

Table 2.2. Potential sources of 'false-positives' when measuring microalbuminuria

---

- Exercise
- Acute fluid intake
- Haematuria
- Menstrual flow
- Urinary infection
- Renal papillary necrosis
- Semen
- Urine collection error
- Laboratory error

---

important are probably posture and exercise, so that it is important to specify the type of urine collection used. For example, the upper limit of albumin excretion rate in an overnight and a 24-hour collection is approximately 10 and 20 µg/min, respectively. Patients with urine positive to Albustix usually have a total protein excretion >350 µg/min of which approximately half is due to albumin. Microalbuminuria, therefore, refers to urinary albumin excretion covering a wide range from 10 to 300 µg/min. Within this range microalbuminuria may be sub-classified according to the various prognostic thresholds of albumin excretion discussed below, and as to whether it is found to be present intermittently or persistently on repeated testing[8,9]. It is important to note that to confidently ascribe microalbuminuria in a diabetic patient to specific glomerular leakiness, non-diabetic renal disease (e.g. pyelonephritis, renal medullary necrosis) and other factors that cause a transitory increase in urinary albumin should also be excluded (Table 2.2).

PROGNOSTIC VALUE AND RISK FACTORS

Four prospective studies collectively showed that microalbuminuria is a powerful predictor of clinical nephropathy in insulin-dependent diabetic patients (Table 2.3). The different thresholds of albumin excretion rate were arbitrarily selected to maximize the detection of patients at risk of developing established nephropathy. Clearly, microalbuminuria bears the worst prognosis the higher the level of urinary albumin excretion and the more persistent the abnormality. 'Incipient diabetic nephropathy' refers to microalbuminuria (>15 µg/min) present on two out of the three occasions over a period of 6 months, in association with an elevated GFR (>150 ml/min), diastolic hypertension (>90 mmHg) and duration of diabetes between 7 and 20 years[6]. Microalbuminuria is very rare in insulin-dependent patients with duration of disease <5 years. It also tends to lose its

Table 2.3. Details of early studies showing prognostic value of microalbuminuria in diabetes mellitus

Study	Viberti et al (1982)	Parving et al (1982)	Mogensen and Christensen (1984)	Mathiesen et al (1984)	Jarrett et al (1984)	Mogensen (1984)
Type of diabetes	IDDM	IDDM	IDDM	IDDM	NIDDM	NIDDM
No. of patients	87	25	44	71	44	204
Follow-up (yr)	14	5	10	6	14	10
No. followed-up	63	24	43	71	42	204
Urine sample	overnight	24-h	resting	24-h	overnight	early morning
Cut-off for albuminuria	30 µg/min	28 µg/min	15 µg/min	70 µg/min	10 µg/min	30 mg/l
No. with DN > cut off	7/8	6/8	12/14	7/7	?	17/76
No. with DN < cut off	2/55	2/15	0/29	3/64	?	7/128
No. died > cut off	3/8	1/8	2/14	0	10/17	59/76
No. died < cut off	5/55	0/15	0/29	0	7/25	62/128

DN = Diabetic nephropathy (clinical proteinuria).

prognostic value for diabetic nephropathy with duration of disease >15 years. The risk factors for the development of microalbuminuria in insulin-dependent patients are poor long-term glycaemic control, hypertension and possibly smoking, dyslipoproteinaemia, elevated GFR and the parental history of renal disease[4,10,11]. Duration of diabetes is a special risk factor, as indicated earlier.

Prospective studies have also demonstrated that microalbuminuria markedly increases the risk of death due to cardiovascular disease in non-insulin-dependent diabetes[7,12]. In these patients microalbuminuria is also associated with the development of clinical proteinuria, but its prognostic power is less with this complication than in the insulin-dependent patient. Epidemiological surveys have also shown that microalbuminuria predicts cardiovascular disease and mortality in non-diabetic subjects[7]. Specific vascular dysfunction and the coexistence of several cardiovascular risk factors may partly account for this very important association of micro-albuminuria.

PATHOGENESIS

Microalbuminuria is due to glomerular leakiness and this may involve the early ultrastructural, blood flow and biochemical changes[4] referred to earlier.

Glomerular Ultrastructure

There is little evidence that a specific ultrastructural change causes micro-albuminuria, although the degree of glomerular basement membrane thickening and mesangial expansion may identify subsets of patients with microalbuminuria who have the worst prognosis.

Hyperfiltration

Hyperfiltration refers to the increase in the renal blood flow and glomer-ular filtration rate seen in diabetic patients. There is good evidence that renal hyperfiltration may aggravate the prognosis of patients with estab-lished microalbuminuria, but there are few data to support its role in for initiating microalbuminuria. There is also continuing dispute as to whether an elevation in blood pressure precedes the development of micro-albuminuria.

Glomerular barrier permeability

Compelling work has shown that the diabetic state reduces the electro-negative charge of the glomerular barrier, attributable to the complex molecule heparan sulphate proteoglycan, by decreasing the activity of an enzyme called *N*-deacetylase. The net effect of this change is to increase the transfer of albumin into the basement membrane and the glomerular ultrafiltrate. Changes in pore size of the barrier are not, however, seen in patients with microalbuminuria, suggesting that the increase in permeability is probably exclusively due to the aforementioned biochemical change.

Conclusion

The pathogenesis of diabetic microalbuminuria is multifactorial (Figure 2.3). It should be noted that a genetic component is probably also involved, as indicated by the familial aggregation of diabetic nephropathy[11] and the well-known finding that only 30–40% of insulin-dependent patients develop significant renal disease[2,5].

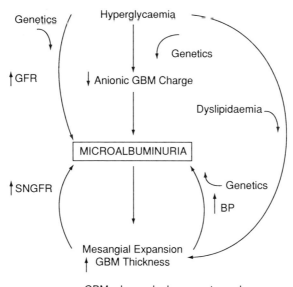

GBM: glomerular basement membrane
GFR: glomerular filtration rate
SNGFR: single nephron glomerular filtration rate
BP: blood pressure

Figure 2.3. Overview of the pathogenesis of microalbuminuria. GBM, glomerular basement membrane; GFR, glomerular filtration rate; SNGFR, single nephron glomerular filtration rate; BP, blood pressure

Prevalence, Incidence and Associations

Cross-sectional studies have reported a prevalence of microalbuminuria ranging from 6 to 60%, but this clearly depends on the threshold of albumin excretion, the selection of patients and the methods and numbers of urine collections employed[8]. For example, urinary albumin excretion is higher in 24 hour and random urine collections than in overnight or early morning samples, and in insulin-dependent diabetics the presence of microalbuminuria is almost restricted to patients with duration between 5 and 15 years. Also, in non-insulin-dependent diabetes microalbuminuria is commoner in those of Asian than of European extraction.

Cross-sectional and case-control studies in insulin-dependent patients have shown that microalbuminuria has a wide spectrum of clinical associations, some of which are shown in Table 2.4[4]. As suggested earlier, the significance of these associations may differ between insulin-dependent and non-insulin-dependent patients[12]. A recently described and most important correlate of microalbuminuria is macrovascular disease (coronary artery and peripheral vascular disease), and this appears to be related to elevations in blood lipids, clotting factors and increased leakiness or permeability of the artery wall[7]. In spite of the many associations of microalbuminuria, a large proportion of the variation amongst subjects remains unexplained, suggesting that in practical terms there are few grounds for establishing a selective screening programme, and this is discussed later[9].

While cross-sectional studies of the associations of microalbuminuria have abounded, the determinants of the progression of urinary albumin excretion have been less extensively studied. An Australian report indicated that in patients with initial albumin excretion rate less than

Table 2.4. The major clinical associations of microalbuminuria in insulin-dependent patients

---

- Early onset of diabetes
- Long duration of diabetes
- Systemic hypertension
- Family history of hypertension
- Retinopathy
- Neuropathy
- Hyperglycaemia
- Male sex
- Smoking
- Dyslipidaemia
- Hypercoagulation

---

30 µg/min the annual incidence of persistent microalbuminuria was 2% for insulin-dependent patients and 4% for non-insulin-dependent patients; insulin-dependent patients who progressed tended to have retinopathy and a longer duration of diabetes and the transition to microalbuminuria was associated with decrease in GFR and increase in blood pressure[5]. A phase of highly variable albuminuria, referred to as intermittent microalbuminuria, may be due to changes in GFR, the significance of which was described earlier. The Microalbuminuria Collaborative Study in the UK reported that in an insulin-dependent patient with albumin excretion rate < 30 µg/min, persistent microalbuminuria also developed at the rate of 2% year and this was dependent on both the initial level of albuminuria, blood pressure and glycated haemoglobin[13]. A 10-year follow-up study of insulin-dependent patients in Portsmouth showed that the most powerful determinant of progression from normo-albuminuria to persistent microalbuminuria was the initial level of glycated haemoglobin and specifically not the level of blood pressure[10]. Once microalbuminuria becomes established the average annual increase in albumin excretion rate appears to rise and ranges from 7% to 20%, but the rate differs widely among patients as shown in studies from Denmark[12]. Variation in the rate of progression at all levels of urinary albumin excretion is probably also determined by complex genetic factors[11].

INTERVENTIONAL STUDIES

This section summarizes the principal interventions[14,15] that have been tested for their effect on microalbuminuria.

INSULIN-DEPENDENT (TYPE I) DIABETES

Glycaemic Control

The Danish Steno I Study carried out over 6 months and the International KROC Study carried out over 8 months concurred that very tight glycaemic control could diminish microalbuminuria. The Steno II Study showed that near normoglycaemia (HbA$_1$ 7.0%) for 2 years prevented the progression of persistent microalbuminuria to clinical proteinuria. A combined analysis of both Steno studies demonstrated that the most pronounced benefit was in patients with higher levels of albuminuria. By contrast to trials in patients with established microalbuminuria, the Norwegian Oslo Study examined the impact of tight glycaemic control (mean HbA$_1$ 8.5%) in patients with a level of urinary albumin excretion around the upper limit of the normal range; after 4 and 7 years continuous subcutaneous insulin infusion achieved a significant reduction in albuminuria compared with no reduction with conventional insulin treatment. The findings of these earlier, small studies have recently been confirmed by the 8-year data from the Swedish Stockholm Study in Sweden and from the large Diabetes Control and Complications Trial (DCCT) in the USA. In the DCCT 1441 insulin-dependent patients were randomly assigned to intensive therapy (continuous subcutaneous infusion or multiple injections) or to conventional therapy[16]. After 6.5 years' intensive therapy that achieved a mean HbA_{1c} of 7% (approximate HbA_{1c} 8%), reduced the development of microalbuminuria by 39% and clinical albuminuria by 54%; there were also parallel improvements in the incidence of retinopathy and neuropathy. The DCCT was a landmark trial that showed that intensive glycaemic control is effective in reducing both the development of microalbuminuria and its progression to clinical diabetic nephropathy.

Blood Pressure

Subclinical elevation of blood pressure is a well-recognized feature of insulin-dependent patients with incipient nephropathy. Because activation of the renin angiotensin alderssterone system induces hyperfiltration and increases pressure with the glomerulus, the major focus on anti-hypertensive agents has been on the so-called angiotensin converting enzyme (ACE) inhibitors. In a 1-year randomized control trial involving normotensive patients with persistent microalbuminuria, a group of French workers reported that Enalapril (an ACE inhibitor) diminished elevated urinary albumin excretion and prevented progression to clinical proteinuria; mean arterial blood pressure was reduced in this study to an average of 85 mmHg. In a randomized control trial of 4-years' duration, another Danish group showed that Captopril (another ACE inhibitor) delayed the development of clinically overt diabetic nephropathy in normotensive, insulin-dependent patients and this has now been confirmed by other studies[17]. ACE inhibitors appear to be better than thiazide diuretics and beta blockers, but there is some dispute as to whether they are superior to calcium channel blockers in the treatment of microalbuminuria.

Dietary Protein

There is experimental evidence suggesting that a high dietary protein intake can damage the kidney by increasing renal blood flow and pressure within the glomerulus. The role of low-protein diets in treating microalbuminuria has not been as well tested as the control of blood glucose and blood pressure. In a small randomized trial lasting only 6 weeks, the Guy's Hospital Group reported that reduction in dietary protein from 92 to 47 g/day resulted in a significant decrease in both microalbuminuria and hyperfiltration independent of changes in glycaemia and blood pressure[18]. In younger patients the effects may be most pronounced in those with elevated GFR, consistent with the previously mentioned mode of action of dietary protein on renal function. Reduction in animal protein instead of vegetable protein may be better in preserving renal function in some patients, but further work is required.

NON-INSULIN-DEPENDENT (TYPE II) DIABETES

By contrast to insulin-dependent diabetes, fewer trials have been carried out in non-insulin-dependent patients[12]. Short-term studies have shown that microalbuminuria may be diminished in patients with newly diagnosed or established diabetes treated with diet alone or diet and oral agents. In the UK Prospective Diabetes Survey in Oxford there was a suggestion in a large group of newly diagnosed patients that dietary treatment alone improved microalbuminuria within 3 months[19]. This effect of a hypocaloric diet may be in part due to the restriction of dietary protein. That improvement in glycaemic control in non-insulin-dependent patients reduces microalbuminuria may be indirectly inferred from the results from the DCCT, but more direct information will be forthcoming from the UK Prospective Diabetes Survey. The relationship between hypertension and nephropathy in non-insulin-dependent patients is less clear than in insulin-dependent patients. A greater proportion of the former are hypertensive and a few short-term trials have shown reduction in microalbuminuria with ACE inhibitors. There is a need for more long-term research studies into the effects of treatment of blood pressure on the incidence and progression of microalbuminuria in non-insulin-dependent patients.

It must be noted that microalbuminuria is only a surrogate end-point for diabetic nephropathy and cardiovascular disease. Although the studies referred to above suggest that microalbuminuria may be amenable to various forms of treatment, no trial has hitherto shown that ESRF or cardiovascular mortality can be prevented. Since the pathogenesis of diabetic nephropathy is multifactorial there is also a case for testing the efficacy of different types of interventions, including inhibitors of prostaglandin synthesis, aldose reductase and growth factors.

PRACTICAL ASPECTS OF THE PREVENTION OF DIABETIC NEPHROPATHY: SCREENING FOR AND TREATMENT OF MICROALBUMINURIA

CRITERIA FOR A SCREENING PROGRAMME FOR EARLY DIABETIC RENAL DISEASE

To justify screening for a particular condition like early diabetic renal disease, the following classical criteria must be fulfilled: the disease should be common and clinically important; it should have an early pre-symptomatic phase; effective treatment should be available for patients who screen positive; the natural history of the latent phase of the disease should be characterized; a reliable and acceptable test should be available with facilities for the follow-up of patient; the cost-to-benefit ratio should be favourable. Screening for early diabetic renal disease by the detection and treatment of microalbuminuria clearly meets most of these criteria. In particular, a recent analysis concluded that screening for microalbuminuria and intervention with anti-hypertensive drugs would have life saving effects and considerable economic saving[20]. Accordingly, the World Health Organization and the International Diabetes Federation have recommended annual screening for microalbuminuria in all insulin-dependent diabetic patients over the age of 12 years and with a duration of diabetes in excess of 5 years.

MEASUREMENT OF MICROALBUMINURIA

Laboratory Methods

These must be specific for albumin and have a lower limit of detection of at least 3 mg/l. This requires the use of immunochemical assays[8]. Immunoturbidimetry using a centrifugal analyser may be the most convenient assay because of its high speed, high precision, inexpensive running costs and requirement for low technical skill. Small analysers are particularly suited for on-line measurements in the diabetic clinic. Urine samples may be stored at $-20\,°C$ for up to 3 months. Assay performance may vary widely and it is therefore recommended that all laboratories belong to a national quality control scheme.

Urinary Collection and Expression of Albumin Excretion

Timed collections are not recommended in clinical practice[8,9]. The most precise and accurate test is the urinary albumin/creatinine ratio (U_A/U_C) in an early morning sample; a random U_A/U_C may be more convenient initially but is less specific owing to the effects of posture and exercise in elevating albumin excretion. Identifying patients with albuminuria in excess of the upper limit of the reference range, i.e. early morning $U_A/U_C > 1.5$ mg/mmol, may yield an unacceptable workload for clinics and it is suggested that initially the programme should aim to detect those with a $U_A/U_C > 3.5$ mg/mmol (equivalent to an albumin excretion rate > 30 μg/min). Thresholds may be regulated according to workload and resources. Measurement of U_A followed by U_A/U_C may be used in combination as a screening test, particularly if there is reason to limit the measurement of U_C. To facilitate follow-up and treatment strategies we recommend that real-time measurements should ideally be carried out during consultations in the clinic.

Side-room Testing

Immunochemical tests such as the latex bead-immunoagglutination test and Micral-test have been developed[8]. These tests only measure urinary albumin concentration and may fail to detect patients with 'true' micro-albuminuria who have a high urine flow rate. We recommend that patients who screen negative by side-room tests should be retested in the laboratory with accurate measurement of U_A/U_C, particularly when there is evidence that the urine is very dilute. In general practice this would require sending additional samples to the biochemistry laboratory of the local district hospital. Training of personnel carrying out these tests is essential.

STRATEGIES FOR SCREENING FOR MICROALBUMINURIA

Selective Screening

Since clinical variables commonly recorded or measured in the diabetic clinic do not confidently predict microalbuminuria, an effective selective screening programme cannot be recommended[9]. However, if screening has to be rationed for any reason it should focus on insulin-dependent patients with early age at onset of diabetes, duration of diabetes between 5 and 20 years, retinopathy, neuropathy, clinical hypertension (BP $> 160/95$ mmHg) and persistent hyperglycaemia (HbA$_1$ $> 12\%$). It must be emphasized that these criteria will not sufficiently increase the sensitivity and specificity of screening to fully justify a selective strategy.

Monitoring Microalbuminuria and Planning Follow-up

Once screening has been initiated, there is a commitment to the follow-up of patients. The most reproducible and convenient test should be used to monitor microalbuminuria. The choice of tests is the U_A/U_C in an early morning (first void) sample. As with first-stage screening, the availability of on-line analysis with the results available at consultation will increase the efficiency of follow-up and treatment. Timed collections, random samples and measurement of urinary albumin concentration alone are not recommended for monitoring purposes[9].

When patients are repeatedly tested for microalbuminuria, many are only found to be intermittently positive. Retesting should aim to identify patients with microalbuminuria present on three consecutive occasions, i.e. persistent microalbuminuria. The retesting interval will depend on the threshold employed in the screening programme to define micro-albuminuria and on the level of albuminuria at initial screening. Use of a threshold to define microalbuminuria is recommended since this will assist clinical decisions. It is suggested that U_A/U_C of 3.5 mg/mmol be adopted to decide whom to follow up with a view to treatment when screening is first introduced in the clinic.

The algorithm in Figure 2.4 is based on data from the natural history of microalbuminuria in insulin-dependent patients in Portsmouth[21,22]. The figure gives retesting intervals based on the level of U_A/U_C in an early morning urine sample at initial screening and a policy to treat patients with microalbuminuria >3.5 mg/mmol on three consecutive occasions[9]. The principle of the algorithm is that the higher the initial value U_A/U_C the more frequently should retesting be carried out with a view to expe-diting treatment. Information on the level of glycaemic control and blood pressure should be taken into account. For example, if the U_A/U_C is <2.5 mg/mmol with an $HbA_1 > 12\%$ and/or a BP of >160/95, the patient should be retested every 6 months. The HbA_1 and blood pressure should be recorded on each occasion that a patient is retested for micro-albuminuria, since this information will not only be useful for deciding further follow-up but will also be important for therapy.

The above recommendations are only provisional and must be validated in a clinical environment. Simpler recommendations have been provided elsewhere, but we consider that these have not been adequately qualified to take account of variation in the individual risk of nephropathy attribu-table to a given level of microalbuminuria. In particular, the recommenda-tion for annual retesting alone overlooks that nephropathy can be rapidly progressive in patients with high levels of albuminuria.

Screening Type II Diabetic Patients

The clinical associations and natural history of microalbuminuria in Type II patients have not been as well studied as in Type I patients. Moreover, the significance of microalbuminuria and the benefits of treatment need to

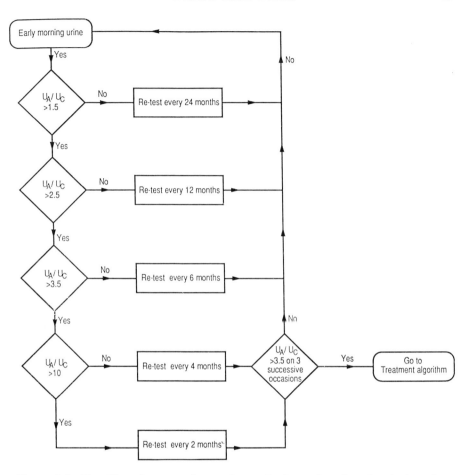

Figure 2.4. Algorithm for screening and monitoring microalbuminuria based on the measurement of the urinary albumin/creatinine ratio (U_A/U_C, mg/mmol) in an early morning sample and a policy to treat those patients found to have $U_A/U_C > 3.5$ mg/mmol on three successive occasions. If the policy is to treat at a lower level of U_A/U_C, re-testing intervals should be shorter[9,22]. The algorithm excludes patients with persistent clinical proteinuria (Albustix > +ve) and elevated serum creatinine

be further established. Routine screening of Type II patients for micro-albuminuria should only be implemented once such information is available from studies currently in progress. It is possible that microalbuminuria may be more specifically and clinically useful as a marker of cardiovascular disease than of nephropathy in Type II diabetic patients[23,24].

TREATMENT

Treatment should focus on patients with persistent microalbuminuria (present on three successive occasions) particularly when the U_A/U_C is rising rapidly[9]. It will need to be individualized, acknowledging that more than one therapeutic option may have to be tried and that the responses among patients may differ[14,15]. Close monitoring of the efficacy of treatment is required by measuring the U_A/U_C at regular intervals. Ideally the U_A/U_C (early morning sample) should be lowered to within the reference range for non-diabetic subjects, i.e. $<1.5\,mg/mmol$. The principal modes of therapy are improvement in glycaemic control, lowering of blood pressure and low protein diets. Use of these in relation to the measurement of microalbuminuria is summarized in the algorithm shown in Figure 2.5. Alternative therapy such as anti-platelet agents and aldose reductors inhibitors is still, however, at the experimental stage. The recommendations for treatment refer specifically to Type I diabetic patients.

Glycaemic Control

Measurement of glycated haemoglobin is important in identifying at risk patients and assessing therapeutic outcome. Treatment should aim to achieve values below four standard deviations above the mean for non-diabetic subjects, e.g. $HbA_1 <7.5\%$ (equivalent $HbA_{1C} <6.5\%$). Control may be improved by conventional insulin treatment or multiple insulin injections[14]. Insulin pump therapy may be considered in selected patients who are highly motivated and well disciplined and for whom the clinic can provide adequate support. Very tight glycaemic control may have drawbacks such as weight gain and unacceptable hypoglycaemia. Attention to regular home glucose monitoring and contact with specialist nurses is important. Given adequate information from their carers, patients will ultimately need to make a choice between the effort and risk of intensified glycaemic control and the risks of developing progressive micro-albuminuria and diabetic nephropathy.

Blood Pressure

Conventional levels of blood pressure used to define hypertension are too high for patients with microalbuminuria. Both the World Health Organization and International Diabetes Federation have recommended early anti-hypertensive treatment of patients with microalbuminuria at blood pressures $>140\,mmHg$ systolic or $>90\,mmHg$ diastolic. It may be useful to employ age–sex matched centile blood pressure charts to define hypertension. Blood pressure should be reduced to <135/85 mmHg (equivalent mean arterial blood pressure 100 mgHg), with due consideration given to age and other complications such as coronary artery disease. A reasonable target would be a blood pressure of 130/80 mmHg with avoidance of hypotension. A conventional sphygmomanometer with diastolic blood pressure readings being recorded at Korotkov Phase V is recommended for clinical purposes. Three measurements of blood pressure should be made in the sitting or supine position, with careful attention paid to identifying postural hypotension particularly in patients with autonomic neuropathy or ischaemic heart disease. Treatment should initially be dietary, with restriction of salt and alcohol and weight loss wherever appropriate. If drugs are required the various options are low dose diuretics (with occasional potassium supplementation), cardiovascular beta blockers, calcium antagonists and ACE inhibitors. Dual or triple therapy may be necessary and plasma electrolyte concentrations should be checked regularly. The efficacy of ACE inhibitors has been well demonstrated in clinical trials and they are considered to be the agents of first choice[17]. Use of ACE inhibitors requires regular checks on electrolytes, particularly for hyperkalaemia, and renal function, which should be undertaken until treatment is stabilized. An alternative therapy may be a calcium antagonist, although the overall evidence for the use of these agents is less convincing than for the ACE inhibitors. Dual therapy may take the form of the addition of a small dose of a loop diuretic to an ACE inhibitor to achieve good blood pressure control. Use of beta blockers and thiazide diuretic needs to take account of hypoglycaemic unawareness, dyslipidaemia and peripheral vascular disease.

Dietary Protein

Patients with microalbuminuria should have specialist dietary assessment to check that protein intake is appropriate and not excessive[9]. A reasonable compromise may be a protein intake of between 12 and 15% of total calories per day or an approximate intake of 1 g of protein/kg body weight per day. Reduction in protein intake should ensure that the patient is receiving an adequate supply of proteins with high biological value and that the diet is not deficient in other essential nutrients. In special cases where other therapeutic options have not influenced the course of microalbuminuria, further restriction of dietary protein or a switch from animal to vegetable type protein may be considered. The above dietary changes can be unpalatable and consequently there may be problems with compliance.

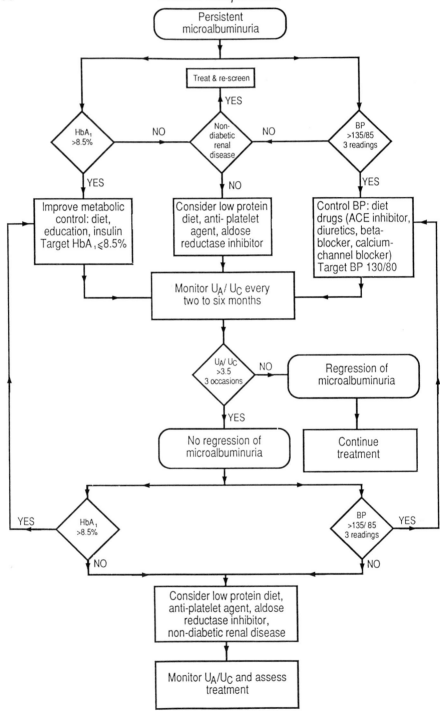

CONCLUSION

Overt nephropathy is probably the most devastating complication of diabetes mellitus. The detection and treatment of diabetic micro-albuminuria offers the hope of preventing nephropathy and its associated problems for a significant proportion of patients. Success depends on the design of an effective screening strategy to detect persistent low-level albuminuria and also of interventional programmes primarily focused on improved glycaemic control and lowering blood pressure. Initially priority should be on insulin-dependent patients, but this may be extended to non-insulin-dependent diabetic patients as the results of ongoing clinical research are published[19,24].

REFERENCES

1 Nathan DM. Medical progress: Long-term complications of diabetes mellitus. *N Engl J Med* 1993; **328**: 1676–85.
2 Viberti GC, Keen H. The patterns of proteinuria in diabetes mellitus. *Diabetes* 1984; **33**: 686–92.
3 Joint Working Party. Renal failure in diabetics in the deficient provision of care in 1985. *Diabetic Medicine* 1988; **5**: 79–84.
4 Watts GF, Shaw KM. The diagnosis and prevention of early diabetic nephro-pathy. In: Raman V, Golper TA (eds), *Preventative Nephrology*. London: Chapman & Hall, 1996.
5 Gilbert RE, Cooper ME, McNally PG, O'Brien RC, Toft J, Jerums G. Micro-albuminuria: Prognostic and therapeutic implications in diabetes mellitus. *Diabetic Medicine* 1994; **11**: 636–45.
6 Mogensen CE. Prediction of clinical nephropathy in IDDM patients. Alter-natives to microalbuminuria? *Diabetes* 1990; **39**: 761–7.
7 Deckert T, Kofoed-Enevoldsen A, Norgaard K, Borch-Johnsen K, Feldt-Rasmus-sen B, Jensen T. Microalbuminuria. Implications for micro and macrovascular disease. *Diabetes Care* 1992; **15**: 1181–91.
8 Rowe DJF, Dawnay A, Watts GF. Microalbuminuria in diabetes mellitus: review and recommendations for the measurement of albumin in urine. *Ann Clin Biochem* 1990; **27**: 297–312.
9 Watts GF, Lowy C, Sonksen PH, Shaw KM. Setting the standards for diabetes care: microalbuminuria. *Practical Diabetes* 1992; **9**: 84–6.
10 Powrie JK, Watts GF, Ingham J, Taub N, Shaw KM. The development of microalbuminuria in insulin-dependent diabetes is determined by glycaemic control and not by blood pressure or angiotensin converting enzyme gene polymorphism. *BMJ* 1994; **309**: 1608–12.

Figure 2.5. Algorithm for treating persistent microalbuminuria (present on three successive occasions). Therapeutic response is based on measurement of the urinary albumin/creatinine ratio (U_A/U_C, mg/mmol) in an early morning sample

11 Seaquist ER, Goetz FC, Rich S, Barbosa J. Familial clustering of diabetic kidney disease. Evidence of genetic susceptibility to diabetic nephropathy. *N Engl J Med* 1989; **320**: 1161–5.

12 Mogensen CE, Schmitz A, Christiansen CK. Comparative renal pathophysiology relevant to IDDM and NIDDM patients. *Diabetes Metab Revs* 1988; **4**: 453–83.

13 Microalbuminuria Collaborative Study Group. Risk factors for development of microalbuminuria in insulin-dependent diabetic patients: a cohort study. *BMJ* 1993; **306**: 1235–9.

14 Mogensen CE. Management of diabetic renal involvement and disease. *Lancet* 1988; **1**: 867–70.

15 Marshall SM. Therapeutic options in early diabetic nephropathy. *Diabetes Revs* 1993; **2**: 6–9.

16 The Diabetes Control and Complications Trial Research Group. The effect of intensive treatment of diabetes on the development and progression of long-term complications in insulin-dependent diabetes mellitus. *N Engl J Med* 1993; **329**: 977–86.

17 Mathiesen ER, Hommel E, Giese J, Parving HH. Efficacy of captopril in postponing nephropathy in normotensive insulin-dependent diabetic patients with microalbuminuria. *BMJ* 1991; **303**: 81–7.

18 Cohen D, Dodds R, Viberti GC. Effect of protein restriction in insulin-dependent diabetics at risk of nephropathy. *BMJ* 1987; **37**: 1641–6.

19 UK Prospective Diabetes Study Group: UK Prospective Diabetes Study 16: Overview of 6 years' therapy of Type 2 Diabetes: A progressive disease. *Diabetes* 1995; **44**: 1249–58.

20 Borch-Johnsen K, Wenzel H, Viberti GC, Mogensen CE. Is screening and intervention for microalbuminuria worthwhile in patients with insulin-dependent diabetes? *BMJ* 1993; **306**: 1822–5.

21 Watts GF, Harris R, Shaw KM. The determinants of early nephropathy in insulin-dependent diabetes mellitus: a prospective study based on the urinary excretion of albumin. *QJ Med* 1991; **79**: 365–78.

22 Watts GF, Kubal C, Chinn S. Long-term variation of urinary albumin excretion in insulin-dependent diabetes mellitus: some practical recommendations for monitoring microalbuminuria. *Diabetes Res Clin Pract* 1990; **9**: 169–77.

23 MacLeod JM, Lutale J, Marshall SM. Albumin excretion and vascular deaths in NIDDM. *Diabetologia* 1995; **38**: 610–16.

24 Watts GF, Jasle M, Cooper ME. The implications of the detection of proteinuria and microalbuminuria in insulin and non-insulin dependent diabetes. *Aust NZ J Med* 1995; **25**: 157–61.

3

Renal Failure in Diabetes Mellitus

G. VENKAT RAMAN

Wessex Renal and Transplant Unit,
St Mary's Hospital, Portsmouth

INTRODUCTION

This chapter will address the problems of renal failure associated with diabetes mellitus, and avoid the aspects of diabetic nephropathy discussed in the earlier chapter. With the exception of accelerated cardiovascular disease in diabetes, renal failure remains the most serious complication in terms of morbidity and mortality. Over the last 20 years the management of diabetic renal failure has made enormous strides, both qualitatively and quantitatively. Up to the 1970s, the onset of renal failure in diabetes mellitus (DM) was considered a more or less terminal complication, and because of the associated vascular and cardiac problems, it was considered a relative contraindication for renal replacement therapy (RRT) or transplantation. That situation has completely altered over the last 15 years, such that currently DM has become the leading contributor to RRT programmes in a number of Western countries, including the USA and Scandinavia. Even in the UK, DM is second only to glomerulonephritis as a cause of end stage renal failure (ESRF) and the gap is narrowing rapidly.

The proportion of European patients with diabetic nephropathy as a cause of ESRF increased from 3% in 1976 to 13.1% in 1987[1]. Within Europe there is considerable variation in the incidence of diabetic nephropathy, with Finland recording a figure of 27.4% of all patients with ESRF in 1987,

Diabetic Complications. Edited by K. M. Shaw
© 1996 John Wiley & Sons Ltd

99% of whom were classified as insulin dependent[1]. In the USA, DM is the leading cause of ESRF, accounting for some 32% of cases for the years 1987–89, with a striking predominance amongst blacks and native Americans[2].

Data from the EDTA Registry show that, between 1985 and 1987, diabetic nephropathy accounted for 12% of end stage renal failure (of just over 66 000 patients). Of all the Type I diabetics who started RRT in this period, 23.5% were aged 15–34, 29% were aged 35–54, 27.5% were aged 55–64 and just under 20% were aged over 65. Of the Type II diabetics 15.7% started RRT within the age group 35–54, 38% within the age group 55–64 and 44% started RRT after the age of 65[3]. The proportion of subjects with diabetes as the cause of renal failure was not different between males and females, though the absolute numbers of male patients affected was significantly greater, with a ratio of 1.4, during this period. Diabetes as a cause of renal failure contributed to approximately 20% of patients with ESRF in northern Europe (Germany and Scandinavian countries), whereas it contributed to only around 13% in southern Europe, Britain and the Benelux countries. According to the EDTA Registry data[4], the survival rates after starting RRT in diabetics at 1, 2, 3, 4 and 5 years were, respectively, 75%, 55%, 45%, 35% and 25% (approximately) for patients who started RRT in the years 1981, 1984 and 1988.

The natural history of diabetic renal disease is evolving continually and progression is constantly influenced by improved treatment modalities. An early report[5] in 1976 suggested a time interval of approximately 18 years between diagnosis of DM (both types) and start of RRT. The interval between presentation to a renal centre and start of RRT was 8 years, and the duration of progression from a serum creatinine of 250 μmol/l to RRT was approximately 4 years.

Current data suggest that approximately 25–40% of Type I diabetics will develop nephropathy between 15 and 25 years after the onset of DM. Amongst Type II diabetics, there is a similar rate of development of this complication, though 5–10% may have nephropathy at the time of diagnosis. Once overt proteinuria has developed, renal failure sets in approximately 7 years later. Typically, once renal failure develops, the progression is relatively rapid, leading to ESRF within 5 years. The average rate of decline of glomerular filtration rate (GFR) is of the order of 5 to 10 ml/min/year, and correlates directly with the blood pressure. However, this progression appears to be modifiable by means of preventive measures. Thus the current advances in management apply to prevention of progression, as much as the treatment of established ESRF.

While diabetic nephropathy remains the major cause of renal failure in diabetics, approximately 10% of diabetics develop renal failure due to other causes. It is therefore important not to be blinkered into the assumption that renal failure in diabetics is always due to diabetic nephropathy. The clues to the presence of non-diabetic renal disease are:

1. The nephrotic syndrome may occasionally be caused by diabetic nephropathy with uncontrolled hyperglycaemia, but is more often due to other diseases like glomerulonephritis. Glomerulonephritis, in particular membranous nephropathy, is the cause of proteinuria and renal impairment in a minority of diabetics. Onset of nephrotic proteinuria, once glycaemic control has been achieved, should raise suspicion of this possibility.

2. The presence of an active urinary sediment points to glomerular disease.

3. Recurrent urinary infections point to the possibility of chronic pyelonephritis.

4. Bilateral small kidneys point to an alternative diagnosis, as typically diabetic nephropathy is characterized by normal to large kidneys.

5. Rapidly developing acute renal failure in a diabetic might point to other conditions such as renal papillary necrosis, which is a recognized complication of diabetes.

6. Patients with diabetic nephropathy are particularly susceptible to develop acute renal failure after administration of radio-contrast media.

PATHOLOGY AND PATHOPHYSIOLOGY

As explained in Chapter 2, the earliest abnormality in diabetic nephropathy is seen in the glomerular basement membrane, with resulting proteinuria. This is first manifested as microalbuminuria for a number of years, after which the proteinuria becomes overt—i.e. detectable by dipstix testing. During the early phases of microalbuminuria, the kidneys are often large and are in a state of hyperperfusion and hyperfiltration[6]. The single nephron GFR, as well as total GFR at this stage are elevated to well above normal levels $(120 \, ml/min/1.73 \, m^2)$, with increased glomerular flow and capillary hydraulic pressure, and diminished renal vascular resistance. As the disease progresses the sustained glomerular hypertension leads to progressive sclerosis of the glomeruli, and there is concomitant development of gross proteinuria. As glomeruli sclerose, the remainder face further increases in blood flow and intraglomerular pressure, thus setting up a vicious cycle. As the glomerular sclerosis progresses further, the total GFR progressively falls (even though the GFR within surviving nephrons continues to increase). When a critical number of nephrons are lost, the GFR rapidly starts dropping below the normal range and leads to progressive renal failure. This whole process is further accelerated by coexistent hypertension. Poor glycaemic control also probably plays an important factor in setting this sequence of events into motion. As mentioned earlier, the combination of these events results in a variable element of ischaemia, which is the final common pathway. Risk factors for progression of diabetic nephropathy include kinetic predisposition, high blood pressure, poor glycaemic control, Afro-Caribbean ethnicity, pyelonephritis.

The natural history of renal failure in Type II diabetes is less well defined, as the diabetes may exist undiagnosed for years, and it is often impossible to identify a date of onset. The clinical situation is further complicated by the frequent coexistence of essential hypertension and degenerative arterial disease affecting the aorta and the renal arteries.

Typically DM is associated with macrovascular disease involving the coronary, cerebral and lower limb vessels; and microvascular disease involving the glomerular and retinal vessels. The classic pathological findings of diabetic nephropathy—nodular and diffuse glomerular sclerosis—were thought to be fairly specific for the disease, associated with specific histochemical abnormalities. It is now recognized that these lesions are simply the expression of diabetic microvascular disease. Indeed, it is worth thinking of the glomerular tuft as nothing more than a specialized portion of the vascular tree, which is particularly suscept-ible to this microvascular disease, and mirrors the more obvious visible retinal abnormalities. Thus, the absence of diabetic retinopathy almost certainly excludes diabetic nephropathy, as the same pathology would be expected to occur at both sites of the microvasculature.

It is now recognized that hypertension is a major contributor to this lesion. Lastly, ischaemia is the final common pathway that results from both these abnormalities, and leads to progressive sclerosis and the associated histological abnormalities. With the increasingly sophisticated use of insulin for glycaemic control and the much improved use of anti-hypertensive drugs, the advanced lesions are now relatively rarely seen.

The structural changes usually seen include an increase in the glomerular volume, accumulation and thickening of the basement membrane, expansion of the mesangial matrix and mesangial cell hyper-trophy. There is an increased synthesis of collagen, laminin and fibro-nectin, with a diminution in the synthesis of glycosaminoglycans and sialoglycoproteins (the latter leading to loss of the anionic charge on the membrane, which allows passage of albumin).

CLINICAL FEATURES

It is beyond the scope of this chapter to go into details of all the clinical features of chronic renal failure. Only those aspects that are particularly germane to DM will be addressed.

1. The duration of DM in Type I diabetics would typically be greater than 15 years, often greater than 30 years. There is a direct relationship between the degree of glycaemic control and the duration before onset of renal failure—the worse the control, the earlier the onset of renal failure. For reasons stated earlier, this relationship cannot be established in Type II diabetics, who may present in advanced renal failure at the very time of diagnosis of DM. Typically, the insulin requirement drops as the renal failure progresses, as the kidneys are a major site of insulin degradation. Males are affected roughly 1.5 times as often as females.

2. Hypertension is almost invariable, and is an early feature, often present by the time proteinuria is detected. It is now considered the most important factor involved in the progression of renal disease in diabetics and the threshold for treatment and target levels have both been dropping successively over the years. There is a genetic component to this hypertension, with a demonstrable abnormality in the sodium–lithium countertransport in the subjects as well as their first degree non-diabetic relatives. Blood pressure is often difficult to control and requires the concomitant use of two or three agents. On occasion, treatment may be particularly difficult when there is associated autonomic neuropathy, causing troublesome postural falls of blood pressure.

3. Proteinuria is invariable by the time renal failure sets in and is usually of the order of 1–3 g/24 hours. Rarely, when the DM or the hypertension is poorly controlled, the proteinuria may reach nephrotic proportions. Microscopy of the urine sediment typically reveals just hyaline casts; the presence of red cells and casts should suggest an alternative diagnosis, such as glomerulonephritis.

4. Hyperlipidaemia is a constant feature, partly related to the degree of glycaemic control. In Type II diabetics, there is a typical constellation of clinical features related to a state of insulin resistance: a marked increase in triglycerides; a modest increase in total cholesterol and markedly low levels of HDL cholesterol. Obesity and hypertension complete the syndrome.

5. Blood biochemistry reveals the usual and progressive rise in serum urea and creatinine. Diabetics, however, have an increased propensity

for hyperkalaemia early in the course of the renal failure. A small proportion of these may be due to pseudohyperkalaemia, which occurs more commonly in diabetics. True hyperkalaemia is sometimes due to the rare syndrome of hyporeninaemic hypoaldosteronism, particularly in the elderly. ACE inhibitors and potassium-sparing diuretics are perhaps the most common cause of hyperkalaemia occurring early in the renal failure. Once renal failure is advanced, potassium retention is, of course, the obvious explanation.

6. Renal osteodystrophy is less common in diabetic renal failure as compared to other forms of renal failure. The classical forms of hyperparathyroid bone disease and osteomalacia are less common than adynamic bone diseases in diabetics.

7. Fluid overload is often seen relatively early in diabetic renal failure compared to other forms. A number of factors contribute to this state—diabetic kidneys have a tendency for salt and water retention, diabetics have a generalized increase in capillary endothelial dysfunction with tendency to interstitial oedema. Last but not least, cardiac failure is common in diabetics because of ischaemic myocardial involvement.

8. Diabetic retinopathy is almost invariably present and leads to variable degrees of visual compromise, which may have major implications for the modality of dialysis treatment.

9. Diabetic polyneuropathy is a relatively common complication by the time renal failure has set in.

10. Renal anaemia due to failure of erythropoietin production is a fairly standard feature, as in all forms of renal failure, but may be a particular problem if there is associated ischaemic heart disease.

11. Neuropathy affecting bladder control may have significant implications for subsequent transplantation.

12. Autonomic neuropathy may produce not only postural hypotension but also gastrointestinal symptoms, which aggravate uraemic gastrointestinal symptoms. Assessment of a diabetic patient with renal failure should be undertaken in an orderly manner, along with a routine plan of investigations, as outlined below.

MONITORING PROGRESSION

There is wide variability in the rate of decline of GFR in patients with diabetic renal failure. On average, once renal impairment sets in, the rate of decline tends to be between 0.5 and 1 ml/minute/month. Serum creatinine is a crude measure of the progression, and the reciprocal of serum creatinine against time is often used to chart the progression. The absolute serum creatinine is obviously influenced by the muscle mass, and as renal failure progresses, malnutrition often sets in in a substantial proportion of patients, with concomitant loss of muscle mass. This can therefore result in a spuriously low serum creatinine, which masks a much greater degree of renal failure. This is a very important fact that is often not appreciated by non-renal physicians.

GFR is most accurately measured utilizing clearance of isotope-labelled DTPA, or by standard inulin clearance. However, these methods are cumbersome and not routinely used in clinical practice to monitor the progression. Creatinine clearance, which is relatively easy to perform, may be used routinely, though it tends to overestimate the GFR.

Whenever a diabetic develops renal failure, a systematic approach should be adopted in terms of clinical assessment and investigations; some guidelines are presented in Tables 3.1 and 3.2.

PREVENTION OF PROGRESSION OF RENAL DISEASE

1. *Blood pressure control.* A large and growing body of evidence suggests that the natural history and progression of renal disease in diabetes can be modified very significantly by meticulous blood pressure control. A diminution in the levels of proteinuria was demonstrated by blood pressure lowering agents belonging to different anti-hypertensive classes[7]. However, there is considerable evidence to suggest that ACE inhibitors confer a particular protection over and above that of simple blood pressure reduction[8]. They have even been shown to be effective and beneficial in normotensive diabetics in terms of reduction in proteinuria[9].

    Meta-analyses of all the relevant studies up to 1992[10,11] suggested that ACE inhibitors reduced proteinuria by 52% (a reduction of 30% at zero blood pressure change), whereas nifedipine actually increased proteinuria by some 21%; diltiazem, verapamil, beta blockers and diuretics reduced proteinuria by 17 to 21%. The findings with the original formulation of nifedipine should not be extrapolated to verapamil, diltiazem or indeed, the newer long-acting dihydropyridines, all of which reduce proteinuria. Thus, ACE inhibitors should be considered the drugs of choice for lowering blood pressure. Evidence suggests that blood pressure lowering should be fairly aggressive and the thresholds for starting treatment should be lower than that for essential hypertension. As a rule treatment should be considered whenever the blood

Table 3.1. Assessment of the diabetic with renal failure

Is the renal failure acute or reversible?
  Consider nephrotoxic drugs—non-steroidal anti-inflammatory agents, ACE
    inhibitors, radio contrast agents.
  Consider acute pyelonephritis.
  Consider renal papillary necrosis or other causes of obstruction.

Could the renal failure be due to something other than diabetic nephropathy?
  Heavy proteinuria or haematuria might suggest glomerular disease.
  Urinary sediment might give clue to glomerular disease or chronic
    pyelonephritis.
  Small kidneys on ultrasonography would point to an alternative diagnosis.
  Evidence of extensive arterial disease elsewhere might suggest ischaemic
    nephropathy.
  Severe or accelerated hypertension would point to hypertensive renal failure.

Can the progression of renal failure be retarded?
  Meticulous blood pressure control.
  Optimize glycaemic control.
  Prompt treatment of urinary infection/pyelonephritis.
  Look for other metabolic problems like hypercalcaemia, hyperuricaemia,
    hyperlipidaemia.
  Exclude any degree of obstructive uropathy.
  Consider introduction of a dietary protein restriction.

Are there other systemic complications of diabetes?
  Ischaemic heart disease.
  Cardiac failure.
  Cerebrovascular disease.
  Peripheral vascular disease.
  Uncontrolled hyperlipidaemia.

Features of chronic renal failure which require treatment?
  Renal anaemia.
  Renal bone disease.
  Fluid retention.
  State of nutrition.
  Uraemic clinical features.

Is the patient eligible for RRT?
  Assessment of quality of life.
  Biological age and general fitness.
  Social situation and family back-up.

Initial modality of RRT?
  Consider primary kidney transplantation (? living related).
  Assess eligibility for HD versus CAPD.
  Allow patient choice if both forms of dialysis appropriate.
  Consider creating arterio-venous fistula in good time—serum creatinine
    $> 500\,\mu mol/l$ (note caveat about muscle loss and malnutrition).

Is the patient eligible and willing to consider transplantation?
  Detailed surgical assessment.
  Explanation of risks and benefits of transplantation.
  Tissue typing and placement on transplant list.
  Consider pancreatic–kidney transplantation in brittle diabetics.

Table 3.2. Routine investigations in a diabetic with renal failure

---

Serial measurements of serum urea, creatinine, sodium, potassium, chloride, bicarbonate.
Serial blood counts.
Initial microscopy of urine sediment.
Quantitation of proteinuria.
Serial measurements of serum albumin, calcium, phosphate, alkaline phosphatase.
Initial screen of serum immunoglobulins and autoimmune profile.
Ultrasound examination of kidneys and outflow tract.
ECG and chest X-ray.
Serum cholesterol, HDL and triglycerides.
Renal biopsy, if doubt of alternative diagnosis.
Doppler scan of vasculature—aorto-iliac segment.
Tissue typing and blood grouping when appropriate.

---

pressure exceeds 140/90 mmHg, and should be considered mandatory if the blood pressure exceeds 160/95 mmHg. Indeed current evidence suggests that proteinuria *per se* is an indication for starting ACE inhibitor therapy, regardless of the actual blood pressure readings. They act synergistically with loop diuretics like frusemide or bumetanide, which should be considered as the standard add-on therapy. Calcium antagonists may be used as second line drugs, preferably avoiding short-acting nifedipine.

Hyperkalaemia is often a limiting factor, which may contraindicate ACE inhibitor treatment. In the minority of diabetics whose renal failure is predominantly ischaemic in origin (more commonly in Type II diabetics, the elderly and those with marked peripheral vascular disease), ACE inhibitors will, of course, lead to a marked deterioration in renal function. In these subjects, calcium antagonists are probably the best drugs to use. Alpha-1 adrenergic blockers are often effective, and additionally have the most lipid-friendly properties. Beta blockers and thiazides may be effective, but are not very popular because of the associated problems. Systolic hypertension may be a particular problem in Type II diabetics, and may be refractory to any form of treatment.

2. There is evidence that *glycaemic control* is of importance in retarding the progression of renal disease, and therefore every attempt must be made to optimize the blood sugar[12]. As a rule multiple insulin dosage is recommended. In obese Type II diabetics, weight reduction would become the most important measure.

3. Treatment of associated conditions like chronic pyelonephritis by antibiotic prophylaxis is of fundamental importance.

4. Dietary protein restriction is of some value in terms of retarding the progression of renal failure. A great deal of research went into this aspect during the 1980s, and there is some evidence that low protein diets (LPD) can reduce proteinuria. While it is recognized that LPD may be effective in a proportion of patients with chronic renal failure, it is not of any benefit in the majority. For this reason LPD has become less popular of late. However, quite apart from retarding the progression, LPD has a definite role in control of uraemic symptoms. The institution of protein restriction has to be balanced against the presence of malnutrition and hypoalbuminaemia. Thus in diabetics who are malnourished for one reason or another (poor intake, urinary protein loss, impaired gut absorption) there is no role for LPD. Furthermore, the application of even more dietary restrictions to an already restricted diabetic diet, is often unpopular and is associated with compliance problems. Nevertheless, once the serum creatinine exceeds 300 μmol/l, it would be reasonable to offer dietary protein restriction of the order of 0.6–0.7 g/kg body weight/day. Patients often report a striking improvement in a sense of well-being once established on LPD.

SYMPTOMATIC TREATMENT

As stated earlier, fluid retention is often an early feature of diabetic renal failure. Loop diuretics should be used, and in refractory cases 250–500 mg of frusemide might be required daily. If the fluid retention is refractory to treatment, it is important to consider instituting fluid restriction, without which there is the danger of pulmonary oedema setting in. The diuresis is potentiated by aldosterone antagonism either by drugs like spironolactone, or ACE inhibitors. The practical limitation to the use of these drugs is the onset of hyperkalaemia. When fluid retention becomes refractory to all measures, dialysis treatment will need to be instituted, even if the biochemistry is relatively acceptable.

Renal anaemia is usually amenable to treatment with recombinant human erythropoietin (EPO). The threshold for starting EPO therapy is arbitrary and in most units it is routine practice to start treatment when the haemoglobin level falls below 7 g/dl. The threshold may be higher if there are concomitant symptoms associated with the anaemia, such as angina. The starting dosage is 2000–4000 units twice a week given subcutaneously, maintenance dose being 100–150 units/kg body weight/week. If haemodialysis treatment has commenced, the EPO can be administered at the end of dialysis. It usually takes between 8 and 12 weeks before the optimal level is reached, with a target haemoglobin of around 11 g/dl. It is important not to exceed a level of 12 g/dl, and the dose should be cut back if that occurs. Some patients can manage with as little as 2000 units a week of EPO, while some may require as much as 12000 units per week. The commonest cause of failure to respond to EPO is iron deficiency, which is simply treated by iron supplementation. Other causes of refractory anaemia include functional iron deficiency, chronic sepsis, occult malignancy, inadequate dialysis, hyperparathyroidism, marrow fibrosis and rarely, aluminium overload.

Other symptomatic treatment measures are:

- Calcium-based phosphate binders for hyperphosphataemia
- Alfacalcidol for osteomalacia (low serum calcium, rising alkaline phosphatase)
- Potassium binding resins for persistent hyperkalaemia
- Quinine sulphate for cramps
- Antihistamines for intractable itching
- Lipid-lowering agents for hyperlipidaemia.

RENAL REPLACEMENT THERAPY

Early results with maintenance haemodialysis (HD) in diabetics were very poor indeed, with a mean patient survival of just 11 months[13]. Refinement of haemodialysis treatment and the advent of chronic/continuous ambulatory peritoneal dialysis (CAPD) in the 1970s transformed the outlook for this group.

Currently, both HD and CAPD are successful and well-accepted forms of treatment of the uraemic state. The choice between the two is a matter of patient preference and availability. Intermittent HD is carried out two or three times a week and the main contraindication to this form of treatment is cardiovascular instability and hypotension. In practice, the limiting factors tend to be dialysis-induced hypotension or angina. The poor state of the vasculature sometimes results in repeated clotting of arterio venous fistulae, but this problem can be overcome by the use of a long-term indwelling vascular catheter. The main problem with the use of vascular catheters is the risk of recurrent septicaemia, usually staphylococcal.

CAPD is generally well tolerated, and is particularly useful where haemodialysis is not tolerated or is unsuccessful, for the reasons mentioned above. The main limitation to CAPD is related to previous abdominal surgery, or the presence of concomitant problems such as aortic aneurysm. Once CAPD is established, it is usually successful. The complication which limits its use is that of recurrent peritonitis. One of the advantages of CAPD is the ability to administer the insulin through the peritoneal route, which often improves glycaemic control. One of the main problems with consideration of CAPD is the visual impairment that is often present in a high proportion of diabetics. However, the problem can be surmounted if there is a spouse or helper who would be prepared to undertake the CAPD to the extent necessary.

The success of kidney transplantation for diabetic renal failure developed rapidly during the 1970s, and became established as the superior form of RRT[14]. Transplantation must be considered the treatment of choice when ESRF sets in. A relatively higher proportion of diabetics are unable to be transplanted due to the associated medical problems such as ischaemic heart disease, advanced generalized arteriopathy, stroke, etc. In the absence of these contraindications, transplantation is very successful in diabetics, as successful as in non-diabetics. The graft survival even with cadaveric donors, often exceeds 80% in the first year, in most units. Living related transplants have a survival of the order of 95%.

A successful transplant is associated with an enormous improvement in the quality of life, the lack of need for dialysis treatment, and the patients usually find their life transformed. Glycaemic control often becomes more difficult, due to a combination of factors—corticosteroid treatment, improved appetite and food intake, cyclosporin A, and efficient breakdown of insulin by the newly transplanted kidney. Cyclosporin A (CyA) is now known to be toxic to the pancreatic islet cells, and tends to aggravate pre-existing diabetes.

The presence of a transplant implies lifelong immunosuppressive treatment and standard 'triple' therapy today consists of a combination of CyA, prednisolone and azathioprine. It is common practice to withdraw one of the three drugs some 3–6 months after a successful transplant, though in many centres they prefer to continue with all three drugs long term. CyA dosage is important, and is titrated according to blood levels— a trough blood concentration of 200–300 ng/ml is considered optimal. Levels higher than 400 ng/ml should not be sustained, as there is a higher incidence of nephrotoxicity. Drugs often interact with CyA, and must be used with great care—e.g. careless introduction of diltiazem can produce a marked increase in CyA levels, leading to nephrotoxicity and even graft failure. The unwanted effects of this long-term immunosuppression include opportunistic infections, and an increased incidence of malignancy after 5 years. Viral warts and squamous cell carcinoma are particularly common and for this reason transplant recipients are advised to avoid exposure to the sun.

Though a successful transplant theoretically only restores renal function, in practice there is a surprising degree of amelioration of the pre-existent non-renal problems such as angina, peripheral neuropathy and other diabetic complications. Part of this may be explained by the rise in haemoglobin back to the normal range. Hypertension remains a major problem, and occurs in the majority of transplanted subjects, both diabetic and non-diabetic. It usually responds to standard anti-hypertensive medication. ACE inhibitors must be used with caution, because of the 5–10% incidence of graft renal artery stenosis. Calcium channel blockers are generally considered the safest in this situation, and have an additional nephro-protective role in the presence of CyA.

Pancreatic transplantation for DM has been slowly gaining popularity over the last 10–15 years. The success rates have been relatively poor compared with other solid organs such as the kidney, the liver and the heart, and for this reason the progress has been tardy. The increased failure is partly related to the technical difficulties in performing the transplant, the problems of dealing with the exocrine secretion, and a relatively higher immunogenicity of the pancreas as a transplant organ. Research is under way into selective islet cell transplantation, but the future is uncertain. For these reasons primary pancreatic transplantation for diabetes remains somewhat experimental and has not gained widespread acceptance. There is a tendency in many units for combined pancreatic and kidney transplantation in diabetics with renal failure, and this is gaining momentum. The one-year survival for pancreatic grafts is only of the order of 50–60%, but surprisingly, the success rates for combined kidney–pancreas grafts ($n = 586$) is slightly better than in kidney only grafts ($n = 1835$)—75% at one year for both, falling at five years to 51% for kidney only grafts, and 57% for kidney–pancreas grafts[15]. Currently efforts are underway in harvesting an adequate number of islet cells and suspending them in a non-immunogenic matrix, which would nevertheless allow the circulating blood/plasma to penetrate to the islet cells, and evoke an insulin response. If successful, this would provide a potentially safe and satisfactory form of pancreatic transplantation in the future.

REFERENCES

1 Brunner FP. End stage renal failure due to diabetic nephropathy: data from the EDTA Registry. *J Diabetic Compl* 1989; **3**: 127–35.
2 USRDS Annual Data Report 1991. Incidence and causes of treated ESRD. *Am J Kidney Dis* 1991; **18**(5) (suppl 2): 30–7.
3 Wing AJ. Causes of end stage renal failure. In: Cameron S, Davison AM, Grumefeld J-P, Kerr B, Retz E (eds), *Oxford Text Book of Clinical Nephrology*. Oxford: Oxford University Press, 1992: 1228–9.
4 EDTA Registry. Report on management of renal failure in Europe, XXIII, 1992. *Nephrology Dialysis Transplantation* 1994; **9** (suppl 1): 10–14.
5 Kussman MJ, Goldstein HH, Gleason RE. The clinical course of diabetic nephropathy. *J Am Med Ass* 1976; **236**: 1861–3.

6 Mogensen CE. Microalbuminuria as a predictor of clinical diabetic nephropathy. *Kidney Int* 1987; **31**: 673–89.
7 Parving HH, Anderson AR, Schmidt UM, Svendsen PA. Early aggressive anti-hypertensive treatment reduces rate of decline in kidney function in diabetic nephropathy. *Lancet* 1983, 1: 1175–9.
8 Bjorck S, Nyberg G, Mulec H, Granerus G, Herlitz H, Aurell M. Beneficial effects of angiotensin converting enzyme inhibition on renal function in patients with diabetic nephropathy. *BMJ* 1986; **293**: 471–4.
9 Marre M, Chatellier G, Leblanc H, Guyene TT, Menard J, Passa P. Prevention of diabetic nephropathy with enalapril in normotensive diabetics with microalbuminuria. *BMJ* 1988; **297**: 1092–5.
10 Kasiske BL, Kalil RS, Ma JZ, Liao M, Keane WF. Effect of antihypertensive therapy on the kidney in patients with diabetes: a meta-regression analysis. *Ann Intern Med* 1993; **118**(2): 129–39.
11 Weidman P, Behlen M, de Courten M, Ferrari P. Antihypertensive therapy in diabetic patients. *J Hum Hypertens* 1992; **6** (suppl 2): S23–6.
12 DCCT Research Group. The effect of intensive treatment of diabetes on the development and progression of long-term complications in insulin-dependent diabetes mellitus. *N Engl J Med* 1993; **329**(14): 977–86.
13 Blagg CR, Eschbach JW, Sawyer PK, Casaretto AA. Dialysis for end stage diabetic nephropathy. *Proc Dialysis Transpl Forum* 1971; **1**: 133–5.
14 Najarian JS, Sutherland DER, Simmons RL. 10 years' experience with renal transplantation in juvenile onset diabetics. *Ann Surgery* 1979; **190**: 487–500.
15 EDTA Registry. Report on management of renal failure in Europe, XXIII, 1992. *Nephrology Dialysis Transplantation* 1994; **9** (suppl 1): 21.

4

Erectile Dysfunction and its Treatment

W. D. ALEXANDER and M. CUMMINGS*

Diabetes Unit, Queen Mary's Hospital, Sidcup, Kent and *Department of Diabetes and Endocrinology, Queen Alexandra Hospital, Portsmouth

It should now be recognized, by all medical practitioners, that not only is erectile dysfunction a common and distressing problem for diabetic men, but usually has a physical cause that it is treatable in the majority of cases by non-surgical means. If all practitioners were to take a degree of interest, advice and treatment could be routinely available.

DEFINITION

Erectile dysfunction (or impotence) is defined as the inability to achieve or maintain an erection satisfactory for sexual intercourse. 'Erectile dysfunction' is currently the preferred term as it encompasses the broader problems of men and provokes less emotion than 'impotence'. In patients who present with 'impotence', it is important to ascertain their perception of the problem for two reasons; firstly, the patient may use the term inappropriately and second, treatment may differ depending on whether the achievement or maintenance of an erection is the main problem.

HISTORICAL PERSPECTIVE

It is only recently that successful physical treatments have become generally available and 'respectable'. Previously, most men with erectile dysfunction would have been either labelled as having psychological problems, or dismissed as having to put up with the problem as a natural function of ageing. If treatment was considered at all, they would likely be referred for sex therapy or to a surgeon, often with a long wait and/or at considerable expense. Psychological treatment for men with diabetes and impotence was disappointing because of the predominantly physical nature of the problem, although it might be argued that treatment was helpful in assisting them in coming to terms with the problem.

Physical treatments of various types have been sought after for many centuries and many have been tried by a few enthusiasts. The problem was not, however, considered very seriously by the medical profession in general until the last 10–15 years.

In the nineteenth century, physical methods might have included relatively useless suggestions such as to rest or to abstain. More aggressive practitioners suggested more active measures such as massage, flagellation or electricity. Galvanic devices producing magnetic stimulation have been in use for a long time and include 'Blakoes Energiser', which is still in use and available.

Vacuum devices and various splints have been in use since the early years of the twentieth century and various surgical techniques have also been tried. Many aids remain available from sex shops, magazines and catalogues.

The formal situation changed dramatically in the 1970s, with an increased understanding of the physiology of erection and increased interest in the problem. The success of new psychological treatments and the Masters and Johnson book *Human Sexual Inadequacy*[1] drew much attention, as did advances in surgical penile implants. Shortly afterwards the work of Virag and then Brindley with intracavernosal vasoactive drugs produced a further major advance[2,3]. This interest also raised the profile of vacuum tumescence devices and as the public became more aware of these treatments so requests for treatment from the medical profession increased. Although in theory treatments were available, people remained reluctant to declare their problem and often the doctor they saw, being equally embarrassed, would neither discuss the problem nor recommend treatment. It is really only in the 1990s that there has been general recognition of the success of treatments, more willingness to discuss the problem and therefore more availability of treatment from physicians both in primary care and specialist units.

It should now be recognized that 80% of men can be satisfactorily treated by non-surgical, non-psychological means, and if all physicians were at least to take a degree of interest, advice and treatment could be routinely available.

PREVALENCE

In the largest study to investigate erectile dysfunction in diabetic males, of 541 patients interviewed, the overall prevalence of the disorder was 35%[4]. The frequency of erectile dysfunction increased with age; 5.7% of diabetic males aged 20–24 years were impotent, increasing to 52.4% in the group aged 55–59 years. This population was re-interviewed five years later[5]. In the group of patients who were originally potent, 28% had subsequently become impotent. Five factors were identified as independently predictive of the subsequent development of erectile dysfunction: age; alcohol intake; initial glycaemic control; intermittent claudication; and retinopathy. Only 9% of those patients who were originally impotent had regained potency, indicating the progressive nature of the disorder.

In the studies of diabetic men, the prevalence of erectile dysfunction has been greater than the above study, ranging up to 75%[6]. Thus, impotence is much more common in the diabetic compared with the non-diabetic population, where the prevalence has been reported to range between 0.1% and 18.4%[7].

WHO TO TREAT

Since erectile dysfunction is common in diabetic men and management can be time-consuming, it is important to identify those patients who are most likely to benefit from medical intervention. Alexander[8] showed that out of 50 diabetic men who completed a questionnaire declaring a problem of erectile dysfunction, only 18% ultimately opted for active treatment. In those patients who spontaneously complained of erectile dysfunction, 88% undertook active treatment. Thus, we would not normally advocate routine screening for the presence of erectile dysfunction, rather intervention should be offered to those patients who seek medical advice for the problem. Most patients are grateful to discuss the problems, however, and this should be encouraged as part of primary care of the diabetic patient.

AETIOLOGY

Table 4.1 lists some of the main recognized causes of erectile dysfunction. It is not uncommon for the aetiology in diabetic patients to be multi-factorial[9,10], for example the diabetic patient with poor glycaemic control, secondary atherosclerotic and neuropathic disease who takes β-blockers or

Table 4.1. Aetiology of erectile dysfunction

Vascular	Arterial insufficiency
	Venous leakage
Neurological	Peripheral/autonomic neuropathy
	Spinal cord lesions
Psychological	
Endocrine	Primary or secondary hypogonadism
	Primary or secondary hypothyroidism
	Hyperprolactinaemia
Renal	Renal failure and dialysis
Pharmacological	Alcohol
	Drugs
Local	Peyronie's disease
	Penile/pelvic trauma
	Phimosis
	Balanitis
	Post-inflammatory fibrosis
	Tumour
	Congenital deformity

Table 4.2. Frequency of aetiological factors in diabetic men with erectile dysfunction[10]

Vascular and autonomic neuropathy	35%
Vascular	35%
Autonomic neuropathy	15%
Psychiatric disturbance	10%
Drugs	5%

other antihypertensive drugs, and becomes anxious because of their lack of sexual performance. The multifactorial origin of the problem is illustrated in Table 4.2 which shows the frequency of aetiological factors in a recent detailed study[10] of diabetic impotent men. A greater frequency of vascular lesions has been observed in insulin-dependent compared with non-insulin dependent diabetic impotent men[11].

A large number of drugs are recognized to cause erectile dysfunction (Table 4.3), usually as an extension of their known pharmacological actions. Thus, drug-induced erectile dysfunction may be reversed by decreasing the dose or discontinuing the drug (see page 80).

It must be noted, however, that the finding of diabetic complications

Table 4.3. Drugs known to cause erectile dysfunction

β-Blockers	Including eye drops. Propranolol possibly the worst, labetolol the least likely to cause erectile dysfunction
Diuretics	Particularly thiazides and spironolactone
Alcohol	
Antipsychotics	Phenothiazines especially thioridazine, lithium. Less likely with haloperidol or pimozide
Antidepressants	Tricyclics and monoamine oxidase inhibitors
Anti-arrhythmics	Verapamil, disopyramide, flecainide, propafenone
Lipid lowering agents	Gemfibrozil, clofibrate
Other hypotensive agents	Hydralazine, methyldopa, prazosin, clonidine
Opiate addiction	
Others	Anticonvulsants, allopurinol, anabolic steroids, baclofen, bromocriptine, cimetidine, ketoconazole, metoclopramide, non-steroidal anti-inflammatory drugs, oestrogens, acetazolamide

which could contribute to erectile failure does not necessarily help in determining treatment, since the problem is often complex and multi-factorial in nature.

ASSESSMENT OF THE DIABETIC PATIENT WITH ERECTILE DYSFUNCTION

An accurate history, careful examination and some simple investigations should elicit the cause of erectile dysfunction and/or appropriate treatment in most diabetic patients without resorting to more complicated investigative procedures. It should be stressed that most of the assessment as to the cause of erectile dysfunction should be part of the regular examination of the diabetic patient. Moreover, erectile dysfunction should alert the care team to the possibility of underlying pathology elsewhere, for example, the patient may also have coronary artery disease as part of widespread vascular pathology which was not necessarily previously detected.

HISTORY

The following questions should be asked.

Initial Useful Questions

What is the problem? Why is it a problem? What is the partner's attitude to the problem? What does the patient hope to achieve as a result of reporting the problem? These general questions will provide an overview of the problem. It may also become clear that, in some instances, the patient will not require any form of medical intervention.

Speed of Onset of Erectile Dysfunction

Psychological erectile failure often presents acutely and is intermittent, whilst organic impotence has a more insidious onset and is complete.

The Presence of Morning, Nocturnal or Spontaneous Erections

The ability to obtain an erection at times other than for sexual intercourse usually implies a psychological origin to the problem. Nocturnal erections have been shown to be resistant to the effects of stress and are not suppressed by psychological means alone[12].

Medical History

Since most cases of erectile failure in diabetic men are of neurological or vascular origin (or both), detailed assessment of the patient's neurovascular systems are required.

Neurological
The nerve supply to the bladder and the penis have the same origin (S2–4). Thus, bladder symptoms may indicate a neurological cause of erectile dysfunction. Evidence of automatic neuropathy elsewhere should be sought, e.g. postural dizziness, excessive sweating, symptoms of oesophageal dysmotility or intermittent diarrhoea. Symptoms of a peripheral neuropathy, e.g. paraesthesia in a stocking distribution may also suggest a neurological aetiology. An enquiry about the presence of symptoms arising from lesions in the cerebral cortex, e.g. cerebrovascular accident, or spinal cord, e.g. demyelination, should also be made.

Vascular
The presence of microangiopathic or macroangiopathic complications in the diabetic patient may suggest that vascular insufficiency is the cause of

the patient's erectile dysfunction. Thus, the patient should be questioned about the presence of angina, intermittent claudication or a past history of ischaemic heart disease, peripheral vascular disease, hypertension, renal disease or retinopathy. Impotence in men who have two or more of the main arterial risk factors (diabetes, smoking, hyperlipidaemia and hypertension) is very likely to be due to artherosclerosis[13].

Glycaemic control
Transient impotence may occur during periods of uncontrolled diabetes and improves following improvement in glycaemic control[14].

Endocrinology
Patients should be questioned about the presence of symptoms which may suggest hypothyroidism (more common in the diabetic patient than in the non-diabetic population), hyperprolactinaemia or hypogonadism.

Current health
Transient impotence may also follow an acute illness[14], e.g. infection or myocardial infarction and this is likely to be psychological in origin.

Drug History

Does the introduction of any drug coincide with the time when impotence was first noted? The patient should be questioned about alcohol intake.

Psychological Assessment

For this purpose, it is best to interview both the patient and partner if they are agreeable. The assessment should focus on five main areas[15]: misconception about normal sexual practice; poor self-esteem and self-image; marital disharmony; and anxiety over sexual performance. The temporal relationship of a specific stress to the commencement of impotence may be elicited.

PHYSICAL EXAMINATION

The following systems should be carefully examined.

Genitalia

The genitalia should be inspected for congenital deformities, balanitis and phimosis. Plaques deposited along the shaft of the penis may suggest Peyronie's disease or intracorporeal fibrosis. The testes should be felt to establish normal size and consistency. Sensation over the penis may be impaired in an autonomic neuropathy. Palpation of each cavernosal artery may suggest adequate blood flow to the penis[16]. A pulsation is best felt by placing two fingers lateral to the midline, midway along the dorsum, with the penis stretched away from the symphysis pubis. Neurological innervation can be tested by assessing the bulbocavernosal reflex (S2–4); pinching the glans should result in contraction of the anal sphincter. Absence of this reflex has been observed in a substantial percentage of men with primary impotence who were unable to ejaculate[17].

Cardiovascular Examination

Evidence of hypertension, ischaemic heart disease, peripheral vascular disease (diminished or absent peripheral pulsations, bruits, poor capillary perfusion) or cerebrovascular disease may indicate a generalized artherosclerotic process contributing to the aetiology. Postural hypotension suggests the presence of autonomic neuropathy.

Neurological Examination

A full neurological assessment should be conducted but in particular, the lower limbs should be assessed for the presence of a peripheral neuropathy. Impaired pain and temperature sensation may be the earliest signs of neuropathy. The presence of autonomic neuropathy can be best assessed by examining the blood pressure response to standing and sustained handgrip, the immediate heart rate response to standing, the heart rate response to the Valsalva manoeuvre and heart rate variation during deep breathing. These simple tests are described in detail elsewhere[18]. Hypothyroidism may be suspected if the reflexes are slow relaxing.

Endocrine Examination

Absence of secondary sexual characteristics suggest hypogonadism. Evidence of hypopituitarism should then be sought to determine if the aetiology is of a primary or secondary nature. There may be evidence of hypothyroidism. Hyperprolactinaemia may be suspected by the finding of gynaecomastia.

Retinal Examination

Evidence of this microangiopathic complication may also suggest a vascular component to the aetiology of the patient's erectile dysfunction.

INVESTIGATIONS

The following tests should be performed by the community health care team.

Assessment of glycaemic control – blood glucose concentration, fructosamine or glycated haemoglobin level.
Assessment of renal function – urine albumin creatinine ratio and plasma creatinine concentration.
Endocrine assessment – testosterone, FSH and LH and prolactin concentrations, thyroid function tests.
Assessment of other diabetic complications – history and examination may suggest other complications which need investigation, e.g. an electrocardiogram or radiological investigation of the pituitary gland.

The following investigations could be performed but are not mandatory prior to initiating treatment.

The Papaverine Test

A test dose of papaverine (or prostaglandin E1) may be injected into the corpus cavernosum. In normal penile anatomy, papaverine induces relaxation of the trabecular cavernous smooth muscles with secondary vasodilation of the penile arteries[16]. The technique is described further in the treatment section of this chapter. Assessment of this method by Virag *et al*[20] showed that all potent volunteers and known psychogenic cases of erectile dysfunction studied had a positive response to intracavernosal papaverine. In another study, this method was found to correlate moderately well with invasive vascular techniques, and of 14 patients with severe arterial lesions and/or vascular leaks, none had a positive response[19]. However, of those patients without severe vascular disease, 50% had a negative response indicating that psychological factors may influence the outcome of this test. Thus, a positive response is helpful since it makes a severe vascular lesion unlikely and demonstrates that intracavernosal injections would be a successful option for treatment. However, a negative response does not contribute to establishing the aetiology nor rule out the use of papaverine as a form of treatment. However, some practitioners may find it useful to perform this test to demonstrate the implications and practicality of the procedure in those patients who wish to pursue active treatment.

Doppler Ultrasound of the Penis

Using a doppler ultrasound probe, it is possible to determine the penile systolic blood pressure. When compared to the brachial artery systolic pressure (the penile-brachial index), this ratio may be useful in determining the presence of vascular insufficiency. A ratio of less than 0.6 is virtually always diagnostic of vasculogenic aetiology[21]. A ratio between 0.6 and 0.91 indicates a variable vascular component while a ratio greater than 0.91 is consistent with normal pelvic haemodynamics[21].

More Detailed Psychosexual Assessment

Referral to a clinical psychologist or psychosexual counsellor may be helpful, particularly in those patients whom an organic cause is unlikely, but do not accept that there is a psychological element to their aetiology. patients with a primary psychological or psychiatric disorder underlying the problem are nearly always likely to require psychosexual assessment.

The following investigations are no longer considered necessary in routine practice. They may be performed in patients referred for possible surgical intervention or for research into the aetiology and future advances in treatment.

More Detailed Investigation for the Presence of Autonomic Neuropathy

In addition to the cardiovascular tests discussed above, the sweatspot test has been used to assess autonomic neuropathy and was the most sensitive test performed in one study[10]. Another simple but sensitive test for autonomic neuropathy is to assess the percentage of iris diameter to which the pupil diameter dilates in darkness[22].

Measurement of Nocturnal Penile Rigidity

Nocturnal erections occur regularly during a typical night of sleep, usually associated with REM[23]. Previously it has been suggested that measurement of penile erections that occur during REM sleep show that in patients whose impotence is psychogenic, nocturnal erections are normal, however those with an organic basis have abnormal erections[24]. It is possible to assess nocturnal tumescence, measuring the maximal increase in penile circumference using a penile strain-gauge and recording onto a portable tape recorder. A simultaneous external occulogram simultaneously records eye movement to determine REM sleep[24]. A more simple estimate of penile rigidity uses a snap-gauge band. When fitted around the penis, the degree of penile rigidity is assessed by the number of plastic film elements that break overnight. In previous studies, normal rigidity causes all three snap-gauges to break while 0–1 breaks suggest organic impotence[25].

Invasive Radiology

Arteriography
Initially a non-selective procedure is performed with introduction of contrast medium into the lower abdominal aorta to establish the extent and severity of disease in the pelvic vessels[26]. If the internal iliac vessels are patent, then selective angiography may be required to demonstrate the arterial supply to the penis.

Cavernosography
This is performed in patients suspected of having venous leaks. This may be suggested in impotent men with a normal penile-brachial index who fail to respond to intracavernosal papaverine[27]. An increasingly rapid infusion of fluid (usually saline) is infused directly into the corpus cavernosum in order to achieve and maintain tumescence. Conventional radiology (or digital subtraction angiography) following a cavernosal injection of contrast medium will then demonstrate any venous leakage.

DISCUSSION AND COUNSELLING

All practitioners should at least be prepared to discuss the problem or let the patient talk about it.

Simple, though perhaps obvious, questions should be a normal part of discussion and are essential for initial assessment:

- What exactly is the problem?

- Why is it a problem?

- What is your partner's attitude?

- What would you like done about it?

These questions are important in determining whether people really have erectile failure rather than some other problem such as:

- False perceptions of normality

- Pain from phimosis

- Peyronie's disease

- Premature ejaculation, etc.

This is important, not only in determining what the problem is, but also whether it will be necessary to refer on to others and if so, to whom. In our experience many men do not wish to pursue physical treatment methods (as currently available) but are pleased to have had the chance to discuss the problem, have it explained and put into perspective[8]. Reassurance or advice about general health and sexual practices is appreciated and many men will come to terms with the problem. Dispelling certain myths about normal sexual practice may be helpful. Dispelling the myth that 'All men are rampant until in their coffins' may reassure a partner who may feel she is no longer desirable, or that her partner is being unfaithful. The myth that 'All women are dependent upon penetrative intercourse for satisfaction' may lead men with erectile failure to feel ashamed, not discuss their problem and completely avoid physical contact with their partner, thereby destroying a relationship unnecessarily, because of performance anxiety. Sex should be for fun. It is not necessarily a performance to be judged against the often unrealistic targets seen, heard or read about, in the media.

The importance of such discussions is to get the problem into perspective. It is inappropriate to refer all men to specialist surgeons or sex therapists if no real problem exists or no treatment is required. It is equally inappropriate to refer a diabetic man with organic erectile failure to a sex therapist as it is to refer a man with entirely psychological problems to a surgeon for the insertion of a prosthesis. It is also rather bizarre that GPs and diabetologists who 'pride' themselves on their holistic approach send their patients to a total stranger as soon as they declare their most intimate problem! *All practitioners should be prepared to provide this level of service.*

PSYCHOLOGICAL THERAPIES

In an ideal world all men should have a multidisciplinary team assessment to include specialist psychosexual advice, but unfortunately this is not possible in practice. All clinicians should therefore have some knowledge of psychological therapies, just as sex therapists will often need to advise and instruct on physical treatments. Although the majority of diabetic men with erectile dysfunction will have an organic basis to their problem, there will be some with primary psychological problems and most with some secondary problems. Physical treatments only restore erections but not necessarily relationships, and there will always need to be some psychological input.

People with overt psychological problems or frank psychiatric disease should be referred for specialist assessment and advice before embarking on the use of physical methods.

There are a large number of psychological therapies of varying complexity involving either the individual or the couple. From the physician's point of view, it is important to have, at least, a general understanding of the principles of 'sex therapy'.

Important aspects of therapies are to identify and agree a number of relevant factors:

- Predisposing factors

- Precipitating factors

- Potentiating factors

- Perpetuating factors.

These should be explored, both as a cue for discussion and decisions on treatment. This will be helpful in improving understanding of the problem, relieving negative thoughts of the patient and directing the physician towards the most appropriate treatments.

SENSATE FOCUSING

The physician may find it helpful to be aware, in detail, of some techniques such as the modified Masters and Johnson approach based on 'couple therapy'[1]. This is a useful and logical treatment, not necessarily in the expectation of restoring erections but at least to restore the concept of physical enjoyment. It should encourage communication, discussion and understanding of the needs, likes and dislikes of the partners and relieve performance anxiety—an important part of the treatment programme.

The suggested programme consists of staged exercises with an agreed ban on intercourse over a set period of time. Half an hour, two or three times a week, should be devoted to these exercises, which involve three phases of sensate focusing:

- Non-genital

- Genital

- Vaginal containment.

Phase 1. In the non-genital phase the couple will caress/stroke and concentrate on enjoyment of touch but not of genital areas.

Phase 2. This allows stroking and caressing to include genital areas. Intercourse should not be allowed to take place even if erection occurs in either of these stages.

The final stage. Prior to allowing normal intercourse, this stage can include vaginal penetration but passively rather than with a view to orgasm or pleasing the partner.

Discussion of techniques such as the modified Masters and Johnson technique should be part of any treatment discussion even if physical methods are to be the mainstay of therapy. Such discussion helps both the physician and the patient to take a broader view of the problem and the purpose of the treatment.

PHARMACOLOGICAL TREATMENTS

There can be no doubt that the major advance in pharmacological treatment has been self-injection with intracorporeal vasoactive drugs (see Appendix 4.1). There are, however, other pharmacological treatments that should be considered.

ALTERATION OF CAUSAL MEDICATIONS

Many drugs have been implicated in causing erectile difficulties and these include alcohol and tobacco (Table 4.3).

The assessment of anyone with erectile dysfunction should clearly include a drug history and consideration of the need for continuing any drugs that might be implicated. Any such drug should be discontinued or changed if possible.

Anti-hypertensive drugs such as beta blockers, diuretics and methyl dopa probably have the most adverse effect. It is worth considering a change to another type of drug such as ACE inhibitors, calcium antagonists or an alpha adrenergic blocking agent. This may be helpful in the younger patient but in our experience is not so effective in the older man who often has underlying peripheral arterial disease.

DRUGS USED FOR TREATMENT

Hormone Treatment

Testosterone has been prescribed for many years but is *per se* ineffective in restoring erectile function to impotent men. It may improve libido, but in so doing may increase frustration if erectile function remains poor. There is therefore no role for its use in men without proven hypogonadism. It is important that testosterone levels are checked, and investigated further if abnormal, because if hypogonadism is proven then testosterone should be used as replacement therapy in its own right.

All men should anyway be screened for carcinoma of the prostate, with a blood test for prostatic specific antigen (PSA), prior to starting testosterone treatment.

Bromocriptine may be beneficial in restoring libido and erectile function in men with primary hyperprolactinaemia after full investigation and assessment of the cause.

Oral Drugs

Yohimbine has been a suggested remedy for erectile failure for many years and there has been much debate about its efficacy. It has also been used in preparations combining it with testosterone. Its effect is probably mediated through its central alpha-2 adrenergic blocking action.

There is evidence that it is more effective than placebo in men with psychological erectile failure, there being a 25% response rate, compared with 5% for placebo[28]. This is not the case, however, in men with organic erectile failure[29].

It may be taken as a regular medication (18 mg daily) or on a prn basis with 6–12 mg taken prior to anticipated sexual activity. Various preparations are available and include Yocon (yohimbine hydrochloride) obtainable by special prescription.

Antidepressants

Although antidepressant drugs have been implicated in causation of erectile failure, they may occasionally be useful in treatment particularly if the problem is associated with anxiety depression. Their action may be related to improvement in mood and relief of performance anxiety, but they may have a more specific effect. *Trazodone*, which has been reported to cause priapism, probably through an alpha adrenergic blocking mechanism, may be tried, either as a course of treatment or on a prn basis of 50 mg 1–2 hours prior to intercourse. Drowsiness may limit its efficacy.

Topical Drugs

Topical vasodilators have been used with only very limited success. A recent study specifically in diabetic men showed disappointing results with transdermal nitrates[30]. Minoxidil cream has also been found to be ineffective[31].

Intracorporeal Self-injection with Vasoactive Drugs (ISIVD)

The injection of intracorporeal vasoactive drugs has been the major advance in pharmacological treatment and is now accepted as one of the

(a)

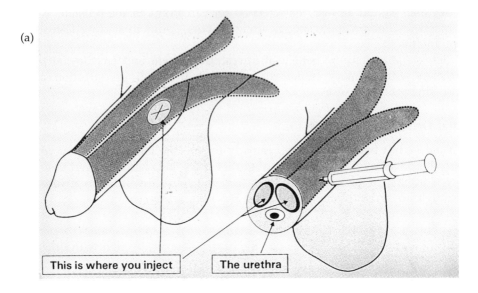

This is where you inject | The urethra

(b)

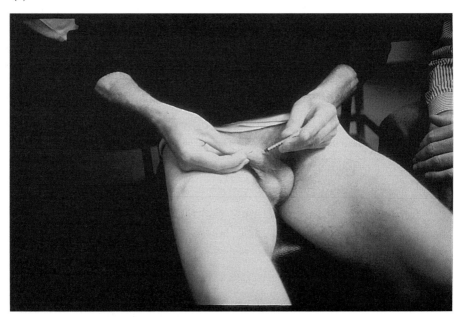

Figure 4.1. (a) The technique of intracorporeal injection. (b) Intracorporeal self-injection

first line treatments for erectile dysfunction. First described by Virag in 1982[2] and subsequently by Brindley[32] it has been increasingly widely used in the last 10 years. It is particularly effective in men with neuropathic impotence and least effective with a vascular cause. It can also be very effective in combination with sex therapy in men with predominantly psychogenic problems. In an ideal world, treatment should always include some psychological input to aid the sexual relationship generally as well as simply restoring the ability to get an erection.

The principle of the treatment is the same regardless of the drug used. When injected directly into the corpus cavernosum the drugs produce relaxation of the smooth muscle and vasodilatation. Provided that the corporeal tissue is responsive and that there is an adequate potential arterial blood supply, erection will ensue (Figure 4.1).

The drugs most commonly used include:

- Papaverine
- Prostaglandin E1
- Papaverine and phentolamine combined.

Papaverine has been the most commonly used drug. It is cheap and stable at room temperature. Either papaverine hydrochloride or papaverine sulphate may be used. Various concentrations are available—we prefer to use 60 mg/ml to keep the volume to the minimum amount. The dose required will vary from person to person between 6 mg and 100 mg. We have found a mean to be about 25 mg. A single vial of 60 mg/ml costs approx £1. Standard disposable insulin syringes/needles can be used. It is not licensed for intracorporeal use and it may be wise to obtain informed written consent from patients before use.

Papaverine/phentolamine combination may be used if there is insufficient response to papaverine alone or large doses are required. A standard dose would be papaverine 30 mg + phentolamine 1 mg.

Prostaglandin E1 is now available as Caverject (Upjohn Ltd) and is the only product actually licensed for intracorporeal self-injection. The recommended dose range is 2.5–60 µg. A single dose currently costs between £7.50 and £10. Initial evaluation suggests that there is a reduced incidence of prolonged erections and of fibrosis at the injection site[33,34]. Relative disadvantages include painful erection in some men, and cost.

INITIATING TREATMENT

It is important that men are carefully instructed on injection technique and doses. It is our policy to provide patients with both pictorial and written instructions (see Appendix 4.1) and to carefully explain the technique with them while they, themselves, draw up and give an initial small dose (6 mg papaverine or 5 µg PGE1) under supervision. It can then be seen by the patient how simple and painless the technique can be. It is rather like initiating insulin therapy, no one is keen to volunteer to give himself or herself injections, but once shown they are surprised how simple it is. Having shown people the technique, it is then our policy to give men instructions for a suggested incremental dose increase, explaining that initially they may not respond, in order for them to find the lowest effective dose. We suggest increases in increments of 10 mg papaverine or 5 µg of PGE1. Such a regime should prevent the occurrence of prolonged erections.

An alternative method used by some is to give serially increasing test doses at separate clinic visits until an effective one is found. We feel this wastes time and that it is inappropriate to equate response in the inhibiting atmosphere of a clinic with that required when sexually stimulated at home.

A third method is to use a large test dose (80 mg papaverine or 20 µg PGE1) to check whether they are likely to be responsive at all. If not, then self-injection therapy is not further considered. This method does carry the risk of prolonged erections and patients need to be observed until the erection subsides and facilities must be available for decompression. It is a method we would suggest should only be considered by specialist urology departments. It has the advantage, if it works, of immediately assuring both patient and clinician, that it will be effective and that erectile function can be restored. Disadvantages are the risk of prolonged erections, it is time consuming and the hospital seating is an inappropriate environment for assessing response.

INJECTION EQUIPMENT

Papaverine can be given with standard insulin syringes/needles. Papaverine and phentolamine mixtures require a larger syringe and separate needle.

PGE1 (Caverject) currently needs to be given with the syringes provided in the treatment pack.

People who find particular difficulty with giving an injection can use one of the autoinjector devices, but we have not found this to be necessary.

FREQUENCY OF USE

It is generally advised to limit use to no more than three times weekly. Clearly the less used the better! Most men will not be using treatment very frequently, in fact many only relatively infrequently but they are still grateful to know that they could produce an erection if necessary.

COMPLICATIONS

Patients should be made aware of possible complications of injection therapy and these include:

1. *Bruising*. Minor bruising will occur in about 25% of people.

2. *Fibrosis and scarring at the injection site*. This can be a troublesome problem and men should be asked to check regularly for areas of scarring. It is not a problem if minor but can produce deformity and pain if more significant. Treatment may need to cease. It has been suggested that this problem may occur less with PGE1.

3. *Infection is extremely rare*.

4. *Prolonged erections*. Prolonged erections have been a much publicized potential problem. It can be prevented by ensuring men use the minimal effective dose. Never should a second dose be given within 24 hours. It is important that men are given instructions on what to do if a prolonged erection occurs. An example of instructions is shown in Appendix 4.2.

5. *Syncope*. Syncope may occur and is usually due to anxiety and not a direct drug effect. Beware injecting men who are very tense and anxious, it is best either to arrange another appointment or at least ensure they are lying down when instructed. Always have some atropine available.

6. Damage to the urethra or dorsal vein may occur if injection is mis-directed into the dorsal or ventral surface rather than the side of the penis.

7. *Split foreskin*. Before embarking on any treatment that may produce an erection ensure that the foreskin is adequately retractable. Men who have not had erections for a long time may have developed a phimosis without being aware of it[35].

Complications are, apart from bruising, a rarity and should be minimized by careful injection technique and careful instruction.

OUTCOME

Adequate long-term outcome studies are lacking. Overall satisfaction rates vary and may be up to 78% in cases of mixed aetiology[36]. We have found a satisfaction rate of 65% in men with diabetes using self-injection treatment for at least 6 months[37]. Dropout rates may be as high as 50%[38], but the reason is not necessarily related to the treatment[39].

VACUUM TUMESCENCE DEVICES

The use of vacuum tumescence devices can provide a safe and effective method of treatment for most men[40,41] and should be discussed and demonstrated as a potential first line treatment (see Figure 4.2).

The vacuum cylinder devices all work on the same principle: A vacuum tube, well lubricated, is placed over the penis with a constriction rubber band placed over the end. A battery or hand operated pump is then attached and a vacuum produced by pumping air out. When sufficient tumescence is produced the band is slipped off on to the base of the penis, the vacuum released and the cylinder removed. The band can safely remain in place for 30 minutes. They do not produce a full erection and the base will remain flaccid with the tumescent penis hanging rather than truly erect, but the result is sufficient for intercourse in 80–90% of men.

There are a number of devices available. Three commonly used include

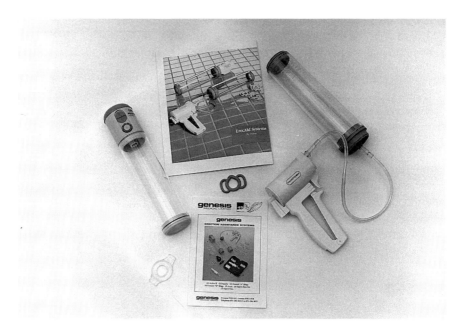

Figure 4.2. Some examples of vacuum devices

ERECAID*, ACTIVE/IMPULSE[†] and RAPPORT**. Prices vary from £119 to £250 depending upon the company and the mode of pump.

Good technique is very important for success and practice may be required. Instructions should be carefully read. Most companies will provide a video instruction tape and also have a telephone helpline to guide people who are having problems. Clinicians should have available demonstration models and videos.

Just as, initially, men may be wary of the idea of injection treatment, so they may be of vacuum devices because of the need for much apparatus and mess which appear to make it rather obtrusive. It is important, therefore, to demonstrate the treatment to people so they can make an informed decision as to which they think will suit them best. Some men may wish to use both forms of treatment. At the least men should be provided with company literature and order forms to give them the option of this form of treatment, as most can be ordered direct without the need for a doctor's consent or prescription.

Expense is a consideration as they are not available on prescription. It may be possible to provide some vacuum devices from hospital appliance departments by local negotiation. Over a long period of time they are very cost-effective compared with injection therapy, since it is only a single, one-off, expense.

UNWANTED EFFECTS

1. *Bruising.* Bruising may occur.

2. *Phimosis.* Significant phimosis should be excluded before recommending use as occasionally restoration of erection may produce tearing of the foreskin.

3. *Ejaculation failure.* This may be due to constriction from the retention ring.

4. *Discomfort.* Some discomfort occurs in most patients but is usually minor. Some patients find the devices rather unnatural, obtrusive and messy. They require a sympathetic and understanding partner.

5. *Cost.* The cost may appear prohibitive and more patients are likely to accept this form of treatment if arrangements can be made for free provision. The companies will refund money to men who are dissatisfied but they still have to pay initially.

---

*Cory Bros Co Ltd, 4, Dollis Park, London N3 1HG.
[†] Genesis Medical Ltd, Freepost WD1242, London NW3 4YR.
**Owen Mumford Ltd, Brook Hill, Woodstock, Oxon, OX20 1PU.

6. *Outcome*. The 'quality' of erection is less normal than that produced by injection therapy and although an erectile state may be produced in up to 100% of men[42], overall satisfaction rates may be as low as 50% and, like other treatments, there is a high dropout rate with time[40,43].

CONSTRICTION RINGS

Constriction rings are available for men who can obtain but not sustain erections and may be considered instead of the complete vacuum device. Such rings have been available for a very long time and are only of limited help.

All practitioners should avail themselves of vacuum device leaflets and order forms and thus be able to provide patients with this form of treatment without the need for specialist referral.

SURGICAL TREATMENTS

Surgical treatments may be considered in three categories: to correct penile abnormalities; vascular surgery; and penile prostheses.

SURGERY TO CORRECT PENILE ABNORMALITIES

- Congenital abnormalities
- Painful conditions such as torn frenulum or phimosis
- Peyronie's disease
- Trauma.

Clearly it is important to establish the presence of such a condition from the history as it is most appropriate then to send the patient to a specialist surgeon/andrologist.

VASCULAR SURGERY

The association between pelvic vascular disease and impotence has been known for a long time[44] but there is much debate about the role of reconstructive surgery. There is no question that it may be useful in men with congenital or traumatic vascular insufficiency and perhaps in men with major vessel disease in whom angioplasty or reconstruction may be of benefit.

In men with generalized arterial disease, microvascular disease, and multiple risk factors, extensive investigation is required to try and ascertain the exact cause of the problem and various microvascular arterial surgery techniques continue to be explored[45]. Such techniques remain largely experimental and most men with such a problem will likely either need to try vacuum devices or have an implanted penile prosthesis.

The role of venous surgery also remains much debated. Various techniques have been used to try and overcome 'veno-occlusive deficits' in men with proven good arterial inflow but inability to sustain erections due to 'venous leakage'. Long-term results from surgery have been disappointing and interest now lies in investigating the cavernosal muscle itself rather than venous channels. Men with such a problem may respond to vacuum devices or require a penile prosthesis.

PENILE PROSTHESES

The implantation of a penile prosthesis remains the mainstay of surgical treatment and with careful selection of patients is very successful in restoring the ability of an impotent man to have intercourse. It is a relatively simple operation that can be performed under general or local/regional anaesthesia.

Most surgeons would reserve the operation for men who have failed to respond satisfactorily to other forms of treatment, including vacuum devices or intracorporeal vasoactive drugs. This most commonly occurs in men with erectile failure from a vascular aetiology but, regardless of cause, some men will require or prefer a prosthetic implant. Careful selection and counselling is important. For efficiency this should be done before referral to specialist surgeons—Cumming and Pryor (1991)[46], for instance, found only 16% of men referred specifically for a prosthesis elected to proceed with the operation after explanation of this and alternative methods of treatment.

Types of Prosthesis

Prostheses are implanted as a pair and most are currently made of a silicone polymer (Figure 4.3). There are three main categories which include: malleable; inflatable; and mechanical.

Malleable prostheses are the cheapest and most reliable. The penis remains erect all the time but can be folded against the abdominal wall or thigh and is easily concealed.

Mechanical and inflatable prostheses contain a mechanism, either intrinsic or attached to the device, whereby it can be kept flaccid or rigid as required.

Complications include infection, mechanical failure, extrusion of the prosthesis, pain and bruising but these are rarely serious, and signifi-

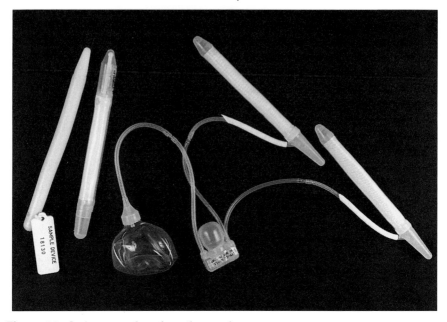

Figure 4.3. Some examples of penile prostheses

cant in less than 5% with adequate precautions and an experienced surgeon[47].

The outcome is high satisfaction rates reported by both patients and their partners[48,49].

CONCLUSIONS

WHICH TREATMENT FOR WHICH PATIENT?

None of the current treatments is entirely satisfactory but most men with erectile failure can have their ability to have sexual intercourse restored by non-surgical means. These include: sex therapy, self-injection with vaso-active drugs, and vacuum devices. Surgical techniques are available for those who do not satisfactorily respond to these.

The choice of treatment will depend upon the individual man or couple and also the attitude and experience of the clinician.

It is often extremely difficult to be sure of the aetiology and it may be irrelevant to initial treatment choice. All men should at least have some discussion and counselling and an explanation and demonstration of the various treatments and an opportunity to try them at home before considering further investigation and surgical referral.

We have found that, after discussion, 30% do not wish to proceed with physical treatments. Of those that do, the majority (68%) prefer to try self-injection treatment[37]. Vacuum devices are a useful alternative and may be suggested as first choice by clinicians not keen to offer self-injection treatment because of their own inhibitions. This is a shame because of the simplicity, more natural effect and effectiveness of injection treatment. Nevertheless, if all practitioners were at least to discuss the problem and offer vacuum devices and provide order forms for their patients, this would considerably increase availability of some treatments.

ORGANIZING LOCAL AVAILABILITY OF TREATMENT

Medical practitioners in all localities are likely to have increasing requests for treatment by men with erectile dysfunction. It is important, therefore, that a local strategy is arranged between primary care and specialist units.

All primary-care physicians should:

- Be aware of the problem, its causes and treatments.

- Be prepared to discuss the problem.

- Have available patient leaflets about impotence.

- Be prepared to offer vacuum device treatment.

- Agree referral guidelines with local specialists for other treatments.

Some primary-care physicians may develop an interest and expertise in sex therapy and/or injection treatment.

A similar degree of interest, knowledge and referral guidelines should be developed by hospital physicians. Referral to surgical clinics could then be reserved for truly appropriate cases, thereby reducing currently long waiting times.

If such a policy were adopted generally, then availability of treatment for this common and distressing problem would be markedly improved.

APPENDIX 4.1

INFORMATION REGARDING TREATMENT OF ERECTILE
IMPOTENCE

Erectile impotence (the inability to obtain or sustain an erection for satisfactory intercourse) is a not uncommon problem in men in general but particularly amongst people with diabetes.

In recent years much work has been done to increase understanding of the problem and there are effective treatments now available.

Treatments available include:

1. *Psychosexual counselling* to overcome psychological factors and for general sex counselling regarding sexual relationships and techniques.

2. *Vacuum devices*   These consist of a vacuum sheath to produce an erection and some have a constricting band to sustain it. They can be successful and acceptable to both partners. They are not normally available on the NHS.

3. *Self-injection therapy*   Injection of drugs such as Prostaglandin E1 or Papaverine into the penis when erection is required may be effective and the technique of self-injection can easily be learnt with specialist help and advice.

4. *Penile implants*   These have been used for a number of years and may be successful. They require a surgical operation and are usually reserved for people who have been unsuccessful with other treatments.

Before embarking on any of these it is important to discuss the problem with your partner (if you have one) and also with your own doctor or specialist. It is important that a full discussion and physical examination are performed to ascertain the likely cause, exclude other conditions of importance and to explain the problem and discuss possible treatments in more detail.

It may be that you are prepared to accept your erection problems and do not wish to proceed to treatment at this stage. This is perfectly reasonable and many couples accept it as a natural inevitability.

The following notes will explain the technique of self-injection treatment.

Dr. William Alexander FRCP.

PROTOCOL FOR SELF-INJECTION

Please follow these instructions.

1. Ensure the room is well lit and you can see what you are doing. You can give the injection sitting, standing, or lying—whichever you find easiest. If you have a tendency to faint then I suggest you inject lying down.

2. Carefully prepare and mix the drugs as per manufacturer's instructions/ video.

3. Fill the syringe with the drug, making sure you draw up all the drug and not just air. Then holding the syringe with the needle pointing upwards make sure you push all the air out. Flick the syringe until the air is at the top and push the plunger gently.

4. *Find the lowest effective dose for you.* This may take some weeks as you must not give a second dose within 24 hours even if the first did not work. This plan is essential to prevent you getting a prolonged erection which can be a serious problem.

   Start with:
   If no good next time try:
   If no good next time try:
   If no good next time try:
   If no good next time try:

   (The maximum dose is the whole 1 ml syringe. If this does not work, please contact me and we will review and perhaps try a mixture of different drugs.)

5. Pull the foreskin right back and hold the tip of the penis firmly with the thumb on the top and the first two fingers underneath. Stretch it as much as possible to one side to get a good view of the side. Insert the needle firmly into the *side* of the fleshy part of the penis avoiding any obvious veins. *Be sure to avoid the undersurface (water pipe) and the top surface (large blood vessel).* (See illustrations.)
   You will feel a slight resistance or grittiness as the needle first goes through the tough outer sheath of the penis. Push the needle right in. Inject the drug. It should go in easily. Undue resistance to injecting the drug means incorrect placement of the needle and you may need to adjust its position or reinsert it.
   After injection remove the needle, press firmly on the injection site for 1 minute to prevent bruising, and massage the penis to spread the drug evenly.

6. Carefully dispose of the syringe, needles and any remaining drug.

7. You should not inject more often than three times a week and never more than once in 24 hours.

8. In the unlikely event of a prolonged erection occurring (more than 4 hours), you must follow the enclosed instruction sheet (Appendix 4.2) and if necessary contact your *local casualty department* taking these sheets of instructions with you.

Self-injection Treatment with Vasoactive Agents—Papaverine/ Phentolamine/PGE1 into the Corpora Cavernosa of Penis

1. The place to inject

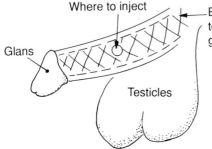

Where to inject

Base; Try and pull all loose skin down towards the base before injecting to get a better view of the area

Glans

Testicles

Injection should be given into the middle of the shaft of the penis. Avoid injecting near the tip (glans). Avoid obvious veins. Inject into the side, not the top or bottom

2. Cross section of penis and injection place

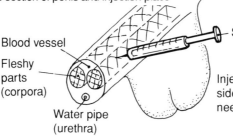

Blood vessel

Fleshy parts (corpora)

Water pipe (urethra)

Syringe and needle

Inject at right angles to side of the penis and push needle right in.

3. Injection place

Blood vessel

Syringe injected right into the fleshy part, avoiding blood vessels, water pipe and any obvious vessels on the surface

Fleshy parts (corpora)

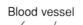

Water pipe (urethra)

Tough outer sheath

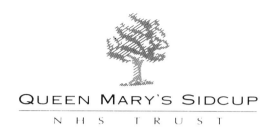

QUEEN MARY'S SIDCUP
N H S   T R U S T

ERECTILE DYSFUNCTION (IMPOTENCE) CLINIC
DEPARTMENT OF DIABETES/ENDOCRINOLOGY

Dear Doctor,
      Re: Mr

Thankyou for referring your patient who was seen in the clinic today and I attach a clinical summary for your records and information.

He has decided to opt for intracavernosal self-injection therapy with Caverject (Alprostadil. Upjohn Ltd.) He has been instructed on technique and dosage and I am happy that he will be able to manage it. He has also been supplied with an instructional video, and leaflet from myself as well as that contained in the product container. I have suggested he start with 2.5 micrograms and gradually increase to find the lowest effective dose.

We would be grateful if you could continue his future management. He has been asked to contact you for further prescriptions and we would be grateful if you could supply these (perhaps on a 10 pack basis, sufficient for at least 3 months, to save him the embarrassment he may feel if having to collect frequent repeat prescriptions). No further appointment has been made for him. He has been told to contact me if he has any difficulties and I would be pleased if you could also let me know if there are any problems with which I can help.

Your patient has been given full instructions on action to take in the event of a prolonged erection so you need not worry about this rare possibility.

If you require any further information please get in touch.

Kind Regards
Yours Sincerely

Dr Bill Alexander FRCP
Consultant Physician

APPENDIX 4.2

INSTRUCTIONS IF PROLONGED ERECTION OCCURS

In the rare event of an erection lasting more than 4 hours and assuming you have tried 'sexual activity', make every attempt you can think of to get rid of it!

1. Try the effect of vigorous leg exercise. Either on an exercise machine or running.

2. Take 2 teaspoonfuls of Sudafed cough mixture.

3. Try ice packs, frozen peas or whatever is to hand.

4. If ineffective try again after a further 1 and 2 hours.

5. If despite these attempts to get rid of the erection it still persists 6 hours after the initial injection *You must go to your local casualty department without further delay even if it is in the middle of the night. It is easy for them to correct the problem if you go early enough. If you delay beyond 8 hours you might require a difficult operation.*

   Take this form and accompanying instructions for doctors with you.

6. Contact me before giving further injections so that we can discuss dosage and technique.

DEAR DOCTOR:

This patient has been instructed by me on the technique of intracorporeal self-injection therapy. He has now developed a prolonged erection unresponsive to the above measures.

I would be grateful if you would follow the enclosed instructions to help him get rid of the prolonged erection or to use your own protocol if preferred.

Thankyou for your attention and I apologise for any inconvenience.

DR WILLIAM ALEXANDER FRCP
Consultant Physician, Diabetes Unit, Queen Mary's Hospital, Sidcup, Kent.

PROTOCOL FOR TREATMENT OF PHARMACOLOGICALLY INDUCED PRIAPISM

Many men with erectile failure are now successfully using intracorporeal self injection therapy with vasoactive drugs. Rarely this treatment may cause prolonged erections and men are asked to attend for detumescence if erection persist beyond 6 hours.

It is essential that this problem is treated urgently.

Suggested treatment protocol

Aspiration

Using aseptic technique, insert a 19–21 gauge butterfly needle (or equivalent) into the Corpus Cavernosum and aspirate 25–50 mls of blood. If detumescence not produced then repeat the procedure on the other side.

If unsuccessful then local alpha-adrenergic medication is recommended.

Alpha-adrenergic intracorporeal injection

- Make up a 200 microgram/ml solution of Phenylephrine in a 5 ml syringe (1 mg total).
- Inject 0.5–1 ml of the solution into one corpora every 5–10 minutes and massage to spread the drug.
- The maximum dose of phenylephrine is 1 mg – (5 ml of the 200 microgram/ml solution).
- If necessary further aspiration of 25–50 mls of blood can then also be tried through the same butterfly needle.
- **Monitor BP and pulse throughout as potential hypertensive crisis can occur.**
- **Caution – if patient is on monoamine oxidase inhibitors**
  – if patient hypertensive
  – if coronary or cerebral artery disease.

If above fails

Urgent surgical referral to urology for further management which may entail a shunt procedure.

APPENDIX 4.3 ALGORITHM FOR TREATMENT OF ERECTILE FAILURE

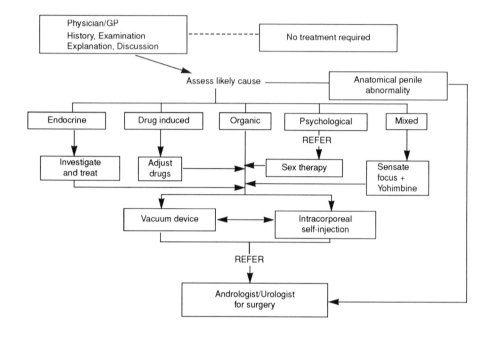

REFERENCES

1 Masters WH, Johnson VE. *Human Sexual Inadequacy*. London: Churchill, 1970.
2 Virag R. Intracavernous injection of papaverine for erectile failure. *Lancet* 1982; **2**: 938.
3 Brindley GS. Cavernosal alpha-blockade: a new technique for investigating and treating erectile impotence. *Br J Psychiatry* 1983; **143**: 332–7.
4 McCulloch DK, Campbell IW, Wu FC, Prescott RJ, Clarke BF. The prevalence of diabetic impotence. *Diabetologia* 1980; **18**: 279–83.
5 McCulloch DK, Young RJ, Prescott RJ, Campbell IW, Clarke BF. The natural history of impotence in diabetic men. *Diabetologia* 1984; **26**: 437–40.
6 Prikhozhan VM. Impotence in diabetes mellitus. *Probl Endokrinol* 1967; **13**: 37–41.
7 Kinsey AC, Pomeroy WB, Martin CE. Age and sexual outlet. *Sexual Behaviour in the Human Male*. Philadelphia: Saunders, 1948; pp 218–62.
8 Alexander WD. The diabetes physician and an assessment and treatment programme for male erectile impotence. *Diabetic Med* 1990; **7**: 540–3.
9 Robinson LQ, Woodcock JP, Stephenson TP. Results of investigation of impotence in patients with overt or probable neuropathy. *Br J Urol* 1987; **60**: 583–7.

10 Ryder REJ, Facey P, Hayward MWJ, Evans WD, Bowsher WG, Peters JR *et al.* Detailed investigation of the cause of impotence in 20 diabetic men. *Practical Diabetes* 1991; **9**: 7–11.

11 Lehman TP, Jacobs JA. Etiology of diabetic impotence. *J Urol* 1983; **129**: 291–4.

12 Karacan I, Salis PJ. Diagnosis and treatment of erectile impotence. *Psych Clinic North Am* 1980; **3**: 97.

13 Virag R, Bouilly P, Frydman D. Is impotence an arterial disorder? A study of arterial risk factors in 440 impotent men. *Lancet* 1985; **i**: 181–7.

14 Podolsky S. Diagnosis and treatment of sexual dysfunction in the male diabetic. *Med Clin North Am* 1982; **66**: 1389–96.

15 Fairburn CG, McCulloch DK, Wu FC. The effect of diabetes on male sexual function. *Clin Endo and Metab* 1982; **11**: 749–67.

16 Cooper AJ. Advances in the assessment of organic causes of impotence. *Br J Hosp Med* 1986; **36**: 186–92.

17 Brindley GS, Gillan P. Men and women who do not have orgasms. *Br J Psych* 1982; **140**: 351–6.

18 Ewing DJ, Clarke BF. Diagnosis and management of diabetic autonomic neuropathy. *Brit Med J* 1982; **285**: 916–18.

19 Buvat J, Buvat-Herbaut M, Dehaene JL, Lemaire A. Is intracavernous injection of papaverine a reliable screening test for vascular impotence? *J Urol* 1986; **135**: 476–8.

20 Virag R, Frydman D, Legman M, Virag H. Intracavernous injection of papaverine as a diagnostic and therapeutic method in erectile failure. *Angiology* 1984; **35**: 79–87.

21 Queral LA, Whitehouse WM, Flinn WR, Zarins CK, Bergan JJ, Yao JST. Pelvic haemodynamics after aortoiliac reconstruction. *Surgery* 1979; **86**: 799–803.

22 Smith SA, Dewhirst RR. A simple diagnostic test for pupillary abnormality in diabetic autonomic neuropathy. *Diabetic Med* 1986; **3**: 38–41.

23 Fisher C, Gross J, Zuch J. Cycle of penile erection synchronous with (REM) sleep. Preliminary report. *Arch Gen Psychiat* 1965; **12**: 29.

24 Hosking DJ, Bennet T, Hampton JR, Evans DF, Clark AJ, Robertson G. Diabetic impotence: studies of nocturnal erection during REM sleep. *Brit Med J* 1979; **2**: 1394–6.

25 Ek A, Bradley WE, Krane RJ. Nocturnal penile rigidity measured by the snap-gauge band. *J Urol* 1983; **129**: 964–6.

26 Hartnell GG. Radiological investigation of impotence. *Br J Hosp Med* 1988; **40**: 438–45.

27 Williams G, Mulcahy MJ, Hartnell G, Kiely E. Diagnosis and treatment of venous leakage: a curable cause of impotence. *Br J Urol* 1988; **61**: 151–5.

28 Reid K, Morales A, Harris C, Surridge DHC, Condra M, Owen J, Fenemore J. Double-blind trial of yohimbine in treatment of psychogenic impotence. *Lancet* 1987; **1**: 421–3.

29 Morales A, Condra M, Owen JA, Fenemore J, Surridge DH. Oral and transcutaneous pharmacological agents for the treatment of impotence. In Tanagho EA, Lue TF, McClure KD (eds), *Contemporary Management of Impotence and Infertility*. Baltimore: Williams and Wilkins, 1988.

30 Close CF, O'Leary H, Ryder REJ. Transdermal glyceryl trinitrate in the treatment of erectile dysfunction in diabetes. *Diabetic Medicine* 1994; **11** (suppl 1): S42, P110.

31 Radomski SB, Hirschom S, Rangaswamy S. Topical Minoxidil in treatment of male erectile dysfunction. *J Urology* 1994; **151**(5), 1225–6.

32 Brindley GS. Cavernosal alpha-blockade: a new technique for investigating and treating erectile impotence. *Br J Psychiatry* 1983; **143**: 332–7.

33 van Ahlen H, Peskar BA, Sticht G, Hertfelder H-J. Pharmacokinetics of vasoactive substances administered into the human corpus cavernosum. *J Urology* 1994; **151**: 1227–30.

34 Schramek P, Dorninger R, Waldhauser M, Konecny P, Porpaczy P. Prostaglandin E1 in erectile dysfunction. *Br J Urology* 1990; **65**(i): 68–71.

35 Alexander WD. Phimosis and treatment for erectile failure. *Diabetic Medicine* 1993; **10**(8): 782.

36 Sidi AA, Reddy PA, Chen KK. Patient acceptance of and satisfaction with vasoactive intracavernosal pharmacotherapy for impotence. *J Urology* 1988; **140**: 293–4.

37 Alexander W. Erectile dysfunction: practicality and evaluation of papaverine self-injection therapy. *Diabetic Medicine* 1994; **11** (suppl 1): S21, P33.

38 Lakin MM, Montague DK, Vanderbrug Medendorp S, Tesar L, Schover LR. Intracavernous injection therapy: analysis of results and complications. *J Urology* 1990; **143**: 1138–41.

39 Armstrong DKB, Convery AG, Dinsmore WW. Reasons for drop-out from an intracavernous autoinjection programme for erectile dysfunction. *Br J Urology* 1994; **74**: 99–101.

40 Ryder RE, Close CF, Moriarty KT, Moore KT, Hardisty CA. Impotence in diabetes: aetiology, implications for treatment and preferred vacuum device. *Diabetic Medicine* 1992; **9**(10): 893–8.

41 Vrijhof HJEJ, Delaere KPJ. Vacuum constriction devices in erectile dysfunction: acceptance and effectiveness in patients with impotence of organic or mixed aetiology. *Br J Urology* 1994; **74**: 102–5.

42 Wiles PG. Successful non-invasive management of erectile impotence in diabetic men. *BMJ* 1988; **296**: 161–2.

43 Bodansky HJ. Treatment of male erectile dysfunction using the active vacuum assist device. *Diabetic Medicine* 1994; **11**(4): 410–12.

44 Leriche R. Des obliterations arterielles hautes causes des insuffisances circulatoires des membres inferieurs. *Bulletin et memoires de la société de chirurgie* 1923; **49**: 1404–6.

45 Sharlip ID. The 'incredible' results of penile vascular surgery. *Int J Impot Res* 1991; **3**: 1.

46 Cumming J, Pryor JP. Treatment of organic impotence. *Br J Urology* 1991; **67**: 640–3.

47 Montague DK. Treatment of erectile dysfunction (editorial). *J Urology* 1993; **150**(6): 1833.

48 McLaren RH, Barrett DM. Patient and partner satisfaction with the AMS 700 penile prosthesis. *J Urology* 1992; **147**: 62.

49 Montorsi F, Guazzoni G, Bergamaschi F, Rigatti P. Patient–partner satisfaction with semirigid penile prosthesis for Peyronies disease. A 5-year follow-up study. *J Urology* 1993; **150**(6): 1819.

5

Diabetic Complications of the Gastrointestinal Tract

D. G. COLIN-JONES

Queen Alexandra Hospital, Portsmouth

Complications of diabetes affecting the gastrointestinal tract, fortunately, are relatively uncommon, but they can be very distressing. Determining whether the symptoms are due to the diabetes is often very difficult in clinical practice as gastrointestinal symptoms are common amongst the general population, and the diabetic may experience these just like any individual. For example, 38% of the general adult population experiences dyspepsia in any six-month period. This is a fairly constant figure. A follow-up postal survey in the UK[1] showed that, while some respondents' dyspepsia settled, others developed it. Furthermore, about 15% of the population have irritable bowel symptoms, with variable bowel actions, distension and a sensation of incomplete evacuation. This has been emphasized by a somewhat reassuring recent large survey of 481 Scandinavian patients with NIDDM and 89 patients with IDDM, who were compared with 635 controls. There was no increase in the number of gastrointestinal symptoms apart from an unexpected slightly lower incidence of gall stones[2]. In managing the diabetic patient presenting with gastrointestinal symptoms, initially, the patient's diabetes should be set to one side and the gut problem dealt with in the conventional way. If no cause can be found for the symptoms, or if there is a failure to respond to standard therapy, then if the problem could be explained by a complication of diabetes, this aspect should be seriously considered.

Diabetic Complications. Edited by K. M. Shaw
© 1996 John Wiley & Sons Ltd

HISTORY AND EXAMINATION

As with everything in medicine, assessing the patient for possible complications of diabetes must begin with a careful history and examination.
One of the crucial things with any set of symptoms in gastroenterology is
how the problem started—was it abrupt, suggesting some infective or
vascular cause, or was it insidious? In addition the length of history is
important, as symptoms of very long duration would suggest that it is
unrelated to the diabetes and has a benign cause. Diabetics are prone to
infections, which require repeated courses of antibiotics. That can lead to
complications such as candidiasis or change of bacterial flora of the colon,
so a careful history should include not only the symptoms, duration, and
how they started, but also whether there were any associated events
around the time symptoms began—such as a chest infection or infected
foot requiring antibiotics, or a myocardial infarct suggesting risk of a
vascular episode.

In addition, knowing whether there are any other diabetic complications
involving particularly the autonomic nervous system is important. Cardiovascular and renal complications tend to antedate any gastrointestinal
problems and so that knowledge of any postural hypotension, renal complications or peripheral neuropathy should be sought on history and
examination. The seriousness of the symptoms also needs to be reviewed,
so that patients who become systemically unwell, with weight loss or
complications such as anaemia, clearly need to be investigated more
vigorously than those with more minor symptoms.

OESOPHAGEAL COMPLICATIONS

Oesophageal motor dysfunction has been found in diabetics, having been
investigated using manometry, barium studies and radionuclides. There
would appear to be a delayed transit through the oesophagus, with
reduced clearance, in up to 35% of diabetics. The oesophageal pressure
waves show an increased frequency of slower peristalsis, with poor
coordination of contractions and decreased lower oesophageal sphincter
pressures[3]. These abnormalities may be entirely symptomless but they
may also be associated with slow eating, and difficulty or discomfort
when swallowing. These motility changes occur frequently in non-diabetic
patients, especially those with gastro-oesophageal reflux and indeed in the
ageing population, so the significance of oesophageal dysmotility in
diabetics is not clear, but it does seem to be more common in diabetics,
especially those with an underlying autonomic neuropathy[4]. However, it
is uncommon to find this as a major problem. NIDDM patients, however,

tend to be overweight, which probably increases the risk of gastro-oeso-phageal reflux disease.

Diffuse oesophageal spasm is the most dramatic of the oesophageal motor disorders and is a condition in which much of the oesophagus goes into intense spasm. Characteristically it affects older people who swallow a larger bolus than usual when eating. There is a gripping retro-sternal pain originating in the oesophagus, they cannot swallow anything, often find it difficult to speak and they break out in a cold sweat. The pain may be intense and it may mimic a myocardial infarct. If they are able to retch back the bolus then they mop their brows and carry on eating, although rather more slowly and with smaller mouthfuls! A barium swallow with bread or marsh mallow is often helpful, and oesophageal manometry may be needed. Treatment is seldom brilliant, with nitrates, nifedipine and occasionally anticholinergic drugs being tried. Rarely a long surgical oeso-phageal myotomy is needed, the circular muscle being cut for much of the oesophageal length—usually, but not invariably, with benefit. Non-specific oesophageal motor disorder is a vaguely defined problem clinically, giving rise to intermittent hold-up in the passage of food, some retro-sternal dis-comfort, which may be severe at times, and waxes and wanes. The causes for these changes are not understood. The myenteric plexus and oesopha-geal musculature appear to remain intact.

DYSPHAGIA

Dysphagia is an important symptom, of great clinical significance, requir-ing careful evaluation. Table 5.1 gives a basic set of questions which will help to separate out the causes. It must be stressed that these patients need investigation, with a barium swallow (with bread or marshmallow if dysmotility is suspected clinically) and upper gastrointestinal endoscopy. Diabetics are prone to cerebrovascular disease and therefore to strokes which can give rise to difficulty with food leaving the mouth—pharyngeal dysphagia. The patient may have difficulty getting the food out of the mouth, or if he or she does then it may be inhaled, leading to coughing and spluttering when the attempt is made. These are very important symptoms, needing careful management and enteral feeding. The patient's cranial nerves need to be examined carefully, the gag reflex checked with a simple probe, and asking the patient to swallow a mouthful of water in the consulting room is often very helpful in determining the pharyngeal (and therefore usually neurological) basis of the symptoms.

OESOPHAGEAL CANDIDIASIS (Figure 5.1)

Diabetics are notoriously prone to infection with *Candida*. This may affect the oesophagus and more rarely the colon. Oesophageal candidiasis often

Table 5.1. Dysphagia

	Helpful specific features	Meaning
Mouth to oesophagus	Does the food leave the mouth/pharynx with ease? Does the patient cough/choke on swallowing?	Probable neurological cause for dysphagia
Within oesophagus i	Recurrent or past history of dysphagia Dyspeptic history Long history Pain on swallowing hot liquids	Probable peptic stricture from longstanding gastro-oesophageal reflux
ii	Steadily progressive dysphagia Weight loss	Probable malignant stricture
iii	Painful obstruction usually relieved by retching bolus back. Patient returns to finish meal	Oesophageal motility disorder
iv	Painful to swallow anything, often acute onset. Recent antibiotics	Oesophageal candidiasis

follows antibiotics, just as with vaginal thrush, and steroids probably increase the risk. Endoscopists now recognize two kinds of oesophageal candidiasis: (1) a very low grade infection with a few white plaques seen in the distal oesophagus which are probably of no symptomatic significance, but likely to flare up if, for example, the patient's diabetes gets out of control or antibiotics are required; (2) the second and more important group is acute oesophageal candidiasis, when florid infection spreads up the oesophageal mucosa, with diffuse white plaques, causing acute dysphagia and especially odynophagia. Any patient who has difficulty with swallowing hot liquids because of discomfort or pain as the hot fluid goes down the oesophagus should have the diagnosis seriously considered. Associated pharyngeal candidiasis should be checked for and if it is present the patient should be treated immediately. Pain on swallowing is an uncommon but diagnostic symptom of oesophagitis, which is most commonly related either to gastro-oesophageal reflux or to an acute infective oesophagitis. Infections involving the oesophagus may be viral, such as herpes (rare), or more commonly fungal—candidiasis. Patients respond dramatically to amphotericin lozenges or Nystatin suspension given frequently during the day. It is a dramatic symptom to the patient and a dramatic one to treat, as in severe cases there may be almost complete

(a)

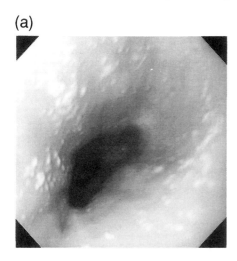

(b)

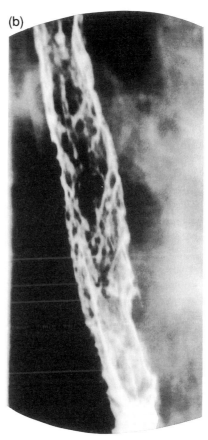

Figure 5.1. (a) Endoscopic photograph of oesophageal candidiasis, showing adherent white plaques attached to the mucosa. Antibiotics had previously been given to this poorly controlled diabetic. Pain on swallowing is the commonest symptom. (b) Radiograph of a barium swallow showing an irregular mucosa due to the adherent plaques. This is a particularly severe example. Minor cases may be missed by this investigation

aphagia because of the pain, which is largely resolved in 48 hours on therapy.

Endoscopy is the best method of making this diagnosis as it shows white plaques adherent to the surface of the oesophageal mucosa, often particularly prominent on the oesophageal folds (Figure 5.1). Brushings can be taken, looking for hyphae. However, endoscopy is not needed in all cases; a typical history justifies treatment immediately.

GASTRIC COMPLICATIONS

Gastroparesis is believed to be a classic complication of diabetes and indeed the term, 'gastroparesis diabeticorum' was first introduced in 1959[5] to describe the considerable delay in gastric emptying that some diabetics experience. Typical symptoms are those of postprandial fullness, epigastric discomfort and distension, nausea, vomiting, heartburn and anorexia. The symptoms fluctuate in severity and usually are insidious in onset. However, they may be exacerbated by an acute ketoacidosis. It is very important to point out that there is a wide range of gastric emptying in normal individuals. Indeed, physiologically, the content of a meal will greatly influence gastric emptying, so that, for example, the emptying of a hypertonic meal (very salty or very sweet for instance) is considerably delayed as most of us know to our cost after an especially heavy meal. There is a large sub-group of non-ulcer dyspepsia known as dysmotility dyspepsia[6] where more than half the sufferers experience objective delay in gastric emptying, particularly of liquids. Thus when it was found that 50% of established diabetic patients had signs of disordered gastric emptying it indicated less that this is a very common complication of diabetes but rather that the range of gastric emptying is wide in the whole population. Only a small minority of diabetic patients actually experience symptoms due to this complication. In the established case there is a strong association between the symptoms of gastroparesis and the development of other diabetic complications associated with an autonomic neuropathy[7]. Curiously there is a great variability in the patient's symptoms. Some patients can be almost entirely symptomless and yet have evidence of considerable delay in gastric emptying, with food residues on a barium meal, despite fasting. Conversely, the patient can have very modest reduction in gastric emptying, with no food residue and yet be intensely nauseated and vomit repeatedly. Severe delay in gastric emptying can occur with other conditions such as systemic sclerosis and amyloidosis.

Vomiting is an important symptom and needs to be assessed by careful history. Vomiting some hours after a meal, with a large amount of food, is a very important symptom of delayed gastric emptying and in the absence of gastric outflow tract obstruction (from lesions such as pyloric carcinoma or stenosing duodenal ulcer) strongly suggests diabetic gastroparesis. Conversely, the patient who retches a great deal (always referred to by the patient as vomiting) but with very little material coming up, has a difficult problem of management but not one of great seriousness in the sense of gastroparesis. It is more related to other triggers which may disturb function, such as uraemia, hypercalcaemia, drug effects, and anxiety. The retching may occur at any time of the day but most frequently occurs first thing in the morning (not uncommonly referred to as 'my early morning sickness'). Care should be taken to look for triggers to this intense nausea/retching as well as checking the stomach itself.

Barium studies tend to show a large stomach with poor peristalsis and delayed emptying. Solid residue may be visualized (Figure 5.2). Radionuclide studies of liquid and solid phase emptying are much more reliable

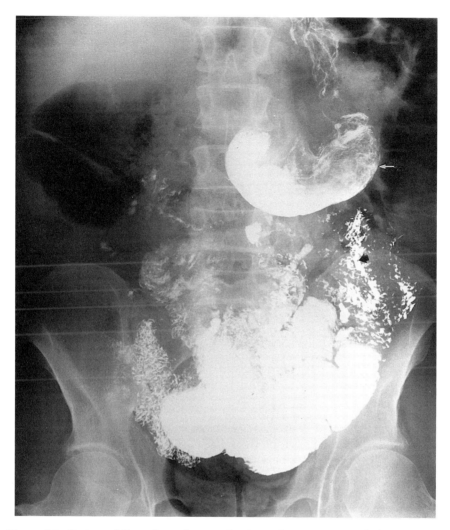

Figure 5.2. Barium follow-through examination of a patient with longstanding IDDM who presented with weight loss, vomiting and diarrhoea. Food residue can be seen in the stomach (white arrow) and flocculation of barium in the jejunum suggested a mucosal abnormality (dark arrow). Coeliac disease proved to be the cause

means of quantifying the rate of emptying and these show striking changes in the severe case (Figure 5.3)[8]. It is particularly the emptying of solids that is delayed. In the severe case phytobezoars may form due to indigestible vegetable matter accumulating in the stomach and becoming

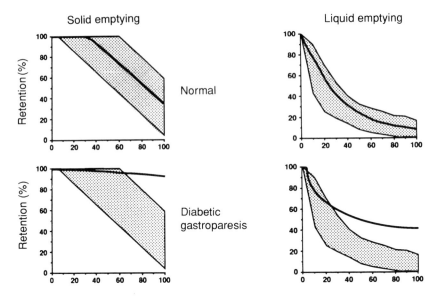

Figure 5.3. Gastric emptying curves for solid and liquid meal components with the normal range (mean ± 2 SD) shown by the shaded area. In diabetic gastroparesis there is marked delay in solid and liquid emptying. (From Horowitz and Dent 1991, reproduced with permission[8])

tangled together so that emptying is impossible. The bezoar can usually be broken up at repeated endoscopy with the help of prokinetic drugs and a liquid diet over a number of days. In such patients it is important to emphasize the need for small mouthfuls, cut up on the plate and well chewed, washed down with plenty of liquid.

Manometric and physiological studies have been undertaken in diabetic gastroparesis, demonstrating a reduction particularly in phase 3 complexes, that is, a loss of good peristaltic contraction waves in the gastric antrum.

The mechanism is not fully understood but there is some similarity with patients who have undergone surgical vagotomy so that it has been suggested that there is demyelination of the vagus nerve in diabetics with gastroparesis[7]. To support this electron microscopic studies have suggested a decreased density of unmyelinated axons in the vagus nerve of such patients. On the other hand the changes found in diabetics are different for liquids where there tends to be a swifter emptying of liquids in post-vagotomy patients. Abnormalities in the gastrointestinal hormones have been found in some cases and are of uncertain significance.

The gastroparesis can be a very major problem in managing the diabetic patient. Because of the delay in emptying it can affect the dietary intake and since, particularly in the early stages, the symptoms and rate of emptying may be variable, it renders control of the blood sugar more difficult to achieve. This is a particular problem bearing in mind that many think that these complications are best managed by tight glycaemic control.

Endoscopy should always be undertaken to exclude an obstructing lesion such as pyloric stenosis, gastric cancer or a duodenal ulcer. If no obvious cause is found for the symptoms a radionuclide study should be undertaken, ideally using both labelled liquid and solid. A barium meal, looking at oesophageal and upper small intestinal function as part of the overall assessment of the patient's motility problem is often useful. A radiologist should specifically be asked to comment on peristaltic activity and the rate of gastric emptying.

TREATMENT

General advice should always be given, such as avoiding hypertonic solutions and fatty meals which delay gastric emptying in everyone. The patient therefore should be encouraged to avoid adding salt to meals, to drink sensible amounts during a meal, to cut up the food well and chew it well. It preferably should have a relatively low fat content with small, frequent meals being better than one large meal in the day. This may mean a change in lifestyle, but the benefits from such simple remedies can often be substantial. Sometimes, however, a prokinetic drug is required, being taken approximately half an hour before a meal. Metoclopramide was the first to be studied. It releases acetylcholine from postganglionic neurones and has anti-dopaminergic properties. This does improve gastric emptying but unfortunately this drug crosses the blood–brain barrier so that it can result in a number of complications, particularly drowsiness, hyperprolactinaemia (with galactorrhoea), and severe Parkinsonian-like complications. Despite these side effects, the drug is often helpful in gastroparesis[7].

More recently domperidone has become available which, as it does not cross the blood–brain barrier, has a better side effect profile. It is a potent dopamine antagonist within the stomach and increases the rate of gastric emptying. Detailed studies in diabetics have not been undertaken. Studies in diabetics have been undertaken with the newer cisapride. It has no anti-dopaminergic activity and works through the cholinergic system, affecting the stomach in particular but with an effect on the oesophagus and whole intestine. It has been shown to increase the rate of gastric emptying and in diabetics substantially improves symptoms[9]. Curiously, correlation between improvement of symptoms and an improvement in gastric emptying is not a good one. Of particular interest is the motilin-like activity of erythromycin. Motilin is a very powerful peptide hormone which dramatically stimulates gastric peristalsis. Erythromycin appears to bind the motilin receptors in the gastric antrum and duodenum leading to a substantial increase in the rate of gastric emptying. Indeed, this property may well be responsible for some of the adverse effects noted in many patients who take this antibiotic. Side effects from this antibiotic are not uncommon, particularly if given intravenously, but there is now a second generation of compounds being developed in which the antibiotic properties have been sacrificed and emphasis been laid on the motilin-like activity. These new compounds offer a very exciting prospect for the future. Lastly, clonidine is an alpha-adrenergic drug which has been found to increase gastric emptying[4]. Anecdotal reports would suggest that it might be helpful. Controlled trials in diabetic gastroparesis are sparse— more are badly needed[7]. The prognosis is unpredictable, worse if the other manifestations of an autonomic neuropathy are prominent, but may remit with the simple measures described and time[10].

COMPLICATIONS AFFECTING THE SMALL INTESTINE

The small intestine is an essential organ, as it is here that the ingested nutrients are absorbed. Problems in its function may arise from *maldigestion*, that is inadequate breakdown of food particles in the lumen of the gut by digestive enzymes; and *malabsorption*, that is inadequate absorption of nutrients through the mucosa. It is an important distinction, because in malabsorption the mucosa will often be inflamed and therefore be more permeable, actually losing nutrients into the lumen, which are then lost. There is, however, sometimes an overlap between malabsorption and maldigestion. For example with bacterial overgrowth of the small gut bile salts are deconjugated, they are then less effective so that there is less bile to dissolve fat, which is therefore less readily absorbed. However, the unconjugated bile salts are more toxic to the upper small gut and a patchy mucosal inflammation may result[11]. As a general principle, due to the nutrient-losing enteropathy, malabsorption is more serious and more difficult to manage than maldigestion.

SMALL INTESTINE—MALDIGESTION

Initially the meal is broken down by the action of digestive enzymes in the lumen of the gut, rendering the nutrients in a small and appropriate form for absorption through the mucosa. This particularly requires pancreatic enzymes. Pancreatic enzyme output may be diminished in some diabetics but is unlikely to be important as most have adequate enzyme secretion. However, chronic pancreatitis can of course present with diabetes. It may not cause pain but rather present with malabsorption or diabetes or both. The diagnosis of pancreatic malabsorption needs to be entertained in any diabetic with diarrhoea, especially if there is no family history of diabetes. A plain X-ray of the abdomen may well show pancreatic calcification, which when present, is invaluable. This is not so much a complication of the diabetes as a complication of the disease that leads to diabetes, namely chronic pancreatitis. The result is a reduction in enzyme output and also a reduction in bicarbonate, so that gastric acid is not neutralized in the duodenum, and the pH in the small intestine falls, which denatures bile salts and may inactivate such small intestinal enzyme as is present. This can lead to severe steatorrhoea and weight loss. It is relatively easily treated by dietary modification with reduction in fat, the use of medium chain triglyceride, pancreatic enzyme supplements in tablet form, and an acid suppressing drug such as an H2 receptor antagonist.

MALABSORPTION

The most important diagnosis to consider here is *coeliac disease*. Coeliac disease is strongly associated with diabetes. Its symptoms are not specific and may therefore be overlooked. There is a strong association with human leucocyte antigens (HLAs)—in particular with HLA-DR3 and HLA-B8. The coeliac population within diabetes is estimated to be 3 to 4%[4]. It is a separate and specific diagnosis rather than a complication of the diabetes, but an illness or deterioration in diabetic control may highlight this inherent defect with increasing symptoms such as weight loss, diarrhoea and anaemia. The albumin is often low. It used to be necessary to take a jejunal biopsy but a very effective screening test is now available—the anti-endomysium antibody[12]. So long as the patient is taking gluten in his or her diet on a regular basis this has turned out to be a remarkably sensitive and specific test for coeliac disease (100% in children and around 95% in adults). If there is any doubt a jejunal biopsy should be taken as the association between coeliac disease and diabetes is a very important one.

These patients then have to take a gluten-free diabetic diet, which is neither easy to do nor is it cheap. But the benefits are very considerable, with improvement in absorption and control of nutrient loss from the inflamed small intestinal mucosa. The diabetic control may become disturbed by the improved absorption when a gluten-free diet is started but is more easily controlled once the patient's mucosa has recovered.

BACTERIAL OVERGROWTH

Bacterial overgrowth presumably occurs because of impaired transit through the gut, allowing colonization with a variety of organisms, particularly *Escherichia coli*, streptococcal species and anaerobes. These organisms have a number of actions, the most important of which is probably the deconjugation of bile salts which renders them less effective and more irritant to the small bowel mucosa, enough sometimes to cause a patchy inflammation in the small intestine, and further adding to the patient's problems[11]. Unconjugated bile salt is not absorbed so well from the terminal ileum (its normal site of reabsorption and recycling). The unconjugated bile salt therefore goes into the colon, which is irritated by its detergent-like property, leading to diarrhoea. There is also probably a toxic factor contributing to the mucosal damage and malabsorption, and hydroxy fatty acids may be formed in the lumen which act like a laxative. This may have a profound effect to reduce absorption, with deficiencies of especially the fat-soluble vitamins, vitamins B_{12}, and K, and increased fluid and electrolyte loss. In theory such effects may contribute to a neuropathy through deficiencies of vitamins B_{12} and E which is of real clinical importance in diabetics with frequent occurrence of neuropathy.

Bacterial overgrowth can be detected using a hydrogen breath test and measuring the rise in hydrogen when a non-absorbable disaccharide reaches the bacteria in the small gut (a shorter time than in normal individuals where bacterial metabolism does not occur until the disaccharide reaches the caecum. It is a very simple test to do. A labelled glycocholic acid test (^{14}C) can be used to determine the deconjugation of bile salts, with the labelled glycine being broken off from the cholic acid, metabolized, and then labelled CO_2 exhaled. A urinary indican is an alternative, in which bacterial breakdown of phenylalanine is absorbed and, as it cannot be metabolized, is excreted as indicans in the urine. It is not as specific as the glycocholic test. Aspiration of jejunal fluid is the 'gold standard' and has the advantage that the organisms can be identified and sensitivities determined. The small gut should be imaged by a barium follow-through examination to assess transit, motility and check for any other disease contributing to the problem.

Ideally treatment should be to eradicate the organisms with antibiotics such as metronidazole or tetracycline given in courses of about ten days to control symptoms. Benefit is usually sustained for long periods after completing the antibiotics, but in more severe cases may prove difficult to control needing long periods on antibiotics and regular changes[11] and should include a trial of ciprofloxacin. If that is unsuccessful a resin such as cholestyramine or cholestid can be tried to bind the bile and reduce its irritant properties on the colon. Should the patient deteriorate on the antibiotic, check the stool for the presence of *Clostridium difficile* toxin. That infection can arise in anyone who has taken an antibiotic and may not be as severe or fulminating as the widely recognized pseudo-membranous colitis.

BILE SALT MALABSORPTION

Bile salt malabsorption arises from ileal disease—typically Crohn's disease but can occur spontaneously in otherwise normal individuals and may affect diabetic patients either because of bacterial overgrowth or spontaneously. It usually responds to a trial with a resin such as cholestyramine.

LACTOSE INTOLERANCE

The brush border of the small intestinal villi contains the disaccharidases, notably lactase. About 6% of the Caucasian population and virtually 100% of the Chinese population do not retain this enzyme into adult life. The gut adapts to this and it is uncommon for milk to induce symptoms in normal individuals. However, there is a potential for other diseases to highlight this enzyme deficiency, with milk-associated borborygmi, distension and loose bowel actions. A lactose tolerance test or hydrogen breath test with lactose will give the diagnosis. Simple dietary exclusion is usually all that is required provided the patient is reviewed for other conditions which have highlighted the lactose intolerance.

DIARRHOEA

Diarrhoea is a common symptom, occurring in up to 20% of the population. Brief attacks which are self-limiting are not uncommon in the general population and do not usually require further investigation but persistent diarrhoea does present a real problem of diagnosis and management. As emphasized earlier, the history and examination are, as ever, vitally important. In particular look for the onset of symptoms and its relationship to other illnesses or antibiotics. Rectal examination and sigmoidoscopy (preferably flexible) with biopsy are essential. Biopsy will sometimes pick up changes of microscopic colitis, not visible to the observer's eye. Stool examination looking for pathogens such as the carrier state for salmonella, persistent cryptosporidiosis, giardiasis should always be undertaken; ideally three samples should be sent.

COLONIC COMPLICATIONS

Any change in bowel habit, particularly in the older patient, requires careful assessment and usually full investigation. Overweight NIDDM frequently have diverticular disease which may be responsible for variable and rather erratic bowel actions. Colonic carcinoma must be excluded by barium enema or colonoscopy. In the majority of cases of diarrhoea the underlying defect is a disorder of motility, with more rapid transit through the gut. The cause is not always apparent. Sometimes it may be due to a change in bacterial flora following antibiotics. The toxin from *Clostridium difficile* should be sought if the stool is liquid. Rarely candidiasis can affect the colon—treatment with oral amphoteracin is usually very effective. These changes in colonic function are not specific to diabetes and not normally regarded as a complication. However, diabetic diarrhoea is a serious problem (see below).

PSEUDO-DIARRHOEA

The passage of frequent, small stools which are usually described by the patient as being diarrhoea but in fact is the passage of small formed stools with a normal faecal weight/volume and consistency is a form of irritable bowel. There is a sensation of incomplete evacuation due to a motility disorder, breaking the faecal material into small amounts which are passed, often with a feeling of great urgency and uncertainty. It is important to assess the faecal volume/weight and correlate that with the number of times the bowels are open. This simple test of collecting all the stools over a 24-hour period is often very helpful.

DIABETIC DIARRHOEA

Diabetic diarrhoea is associated with longstanding IDDM and is strongly associated with an autonomic neuropathy and other diabetic complications, so that if the diagnosis is being considered, evidence of an autonomic neuropathy should be sought[13]. Gastroparesis is quite a common associated gastrointestinal problem. The stools are usually watery and disturb the patient at night. This night-time diarrhoea is a very important feature, pointing towards an organic cause for the diarrhoea and, in the diabetic, very suggestive that this is diabetic diarrhoea[14]. Pain is not a feature, but there is urgency of defecation and sometimes incontinence, particularly at night. The management is outlined in Figure 5.5, which is in the form of an algorithm. When advising diabetics with diarrhoea, first exclude specific causes. Bacterial overgrowth forms a significant group within so-called diabetic diarrhoea and should be investigated and treated

Table 5.2. Causes of diarrhoea in diabetics

Small intestine	–	malabsorption (mucosal disease such as coeliac disease)
	–	maldigestion (lack of digestive enzyme such as in chronic pancreatitis)
	–	bacterial overgrowth
	–	bile salt malabsorption
	–	coeliac disease (gluten sensitive)
	–	lactose intolerance
Colon	–	motility
	–	change in bacterial flora, especially antibiotic induced
	–	anorectal dysfunction
Both small and large intestine	–	secretory diarrhoea
Pseudo-diarrhoea	–	passage of frequent small stools, but normal faecal volume (irritable bowel)

as outlined above. True diabetic diarrhoea is where no obvious cause can be found for the diarrhoea and the patient has evidence in other systems of an autonomic neuropathy. It may be very difficult indeed to treat[15] (see below).

BOTH SMALL AND LARGE INTESTINES

The majority of cases of diarrhoea are due to swift transit through the gut, a motility problem. Occasionally, however, the diarrhoea may be *secretory*. (The classic example of this is cholera, in which a toxin produced by the *Vibrio cholerae* causes secretion of intestinal fluid which overwhelms any absorptive capacity of small and large intestine and results in watery diarrhoea.) Severe cases of diabetic diarrhoea may experience this secretory type of diarrhoea. The mechanism is unknown but it is serious, causing great disability and being very difficult to control. The hallmark of it is a high volume fluid stool which may lead to incontinence. It is diagnosed by fasting the patient for 48 hours (with intravenous feeding) and measuring the stool volume, which diminishes little despite the absence of a food stimulus to gut function. Bacterial overgrowth and an autonomic neuropathy are contributors to this intractable problem. Somatostatin has recently been shown to be of some help in these individuals[16].

INCONTINENCE

Incontinence is a not uncommon problem in the general population. It occurs also in the diabetic and causes great distress, varying in severity from a little faecal soiling with the passage of flatus to profound loss of control. Many patients find this so distressing that it is quite difficult to get an accurate history and anxiety may well play a role in perpetuating or worsening the symptoms—which is not surprising for anyone wishing to lead an active and normal life. The history of night-time incontinence, with fluid stools and lack of awareness of impending defecation are all important clues, as are other features of an autonomic neuropathy. Rectal examination must include an anal reflex, in which the skin adjacent to the anal canal is scratched with a needle, causing reflex visible contraction of the external anal sphincter. This is often lost in an autonomic neuropathy or where damage has occurred to the pudendal nerve at difficult childbirth. The index finger is then inserted and a normal rectal examination carried out. The consistency of any faeces should be noted if present. The anal tone must then be assessed in the (hopefully) relaxed state, after which the patient should be asked to squeeze the anal canal as if to prevent passage of stool. Distinction must be made between closure of the external anal sphincter and the levator ani, which is the muscle of the pelvic floor. Some patients, especially younger ones, to compensate for weakness of the anal sphincter, develop the technique of tightening the pelvic floor, which can occlude the anal canal by lateral pressure. The levator ani causes an acute anorectal angle. Many patients who are incontinent will have lost the anorectal angle, which is an important part of the continent mechanism (Figure 5.4). If the angle is lost then the rectum points straight down on to the lumen of the anal canal and control depends solely upon the sphincter. If there is a strong pelvic floor and a good angle then there is much less dependence on the sphincter. These things can all readily be assessed by rectal examination. In women who have had difficult childbirth there may be a pudendal nerve defect contributing to these symptoms which can be indistinguishable from incontinence associated with diabetes, except for other evidence of a neuropathy. It is important to assess the colon fully with sigmoidoscopy and a barium enema/colonoscopy, looking for function, loss of haustra, tendency to spasm, which may be contributing to the symptoms. Defecography may help assess the continence mechanism. In specialist centres measurement of rectal sensation by balloon and anorectal manometry may contribute. A liquid stool may be difficult to retain whereas a formed stool may present no problems to the patient, so a key aim in therapy is to achieve a formed stool. Pelvic floor exercises can sometimes help by strengthening the levator ani. Many of these patients are overweight and regular exercise does not come easily. Furthermore, a number of women will have pudendal nerve lesions which may not be related to their diabetes, and these reduce the patients' ability to help strengthen the pelvic floor. None the less, bio-feedback by skilled counselling can be

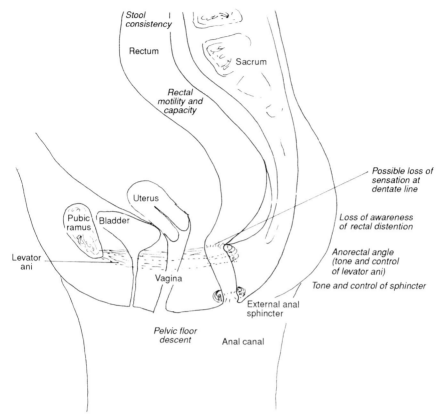

Figure 5.4. The causes of incontinence are numerous affecting many people not just diabetics. This is a schematic illustration of the pelvic anatomy (normal print) and potential causes of incontinence (italics)

helpful in anal dysfunction. Implantable mechanical devices have been tried but often seem to be unsuccessful—partly because of the loss of the anorectal angle in so many of these patients.

TREATMENT

The key to successful management lies in establishing the cause when this is possible, such as enteropathogens, colonic disease, coeliac disease, pancreatic malabsorption and laxative abuse (Figure 5.5). Thus pancreatic enzyme supplements, a gluten-free diet, are dramatically effective in the

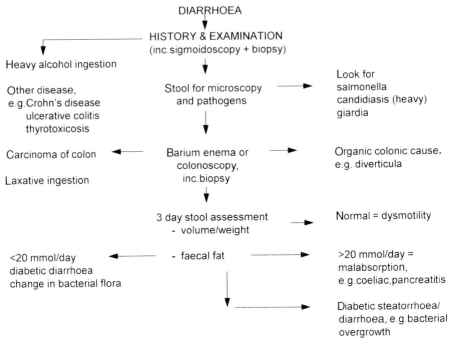

Figure 5.5. Causes and treatment of diarrhoea

appropriate cases. Bacterial overgrowth initially should be treated with antibiotics such as tetracycline or metronidazole, with a benefit from a 10-day course often lasting many weeks. A resin such as cholestyramine or colestipol should be considered if the patient is requiring too frequent antibiotics or is not responding. In the dysmotility patients conventional anti-diarrhoeals such as loperamide or codeine can often lead to an over-swing and constipation. An antispasmodic such as mebeverine, alverine or dicyclomine should be considered. A bulking agent such as ispaghula is quite often helpful by its water-absorbing capacity. Clonidine, an alpha-2 adrenergic agonist, may influence enterocyte function through the adrenergic system where there is an autonomic neuropathy, to reduce fluid output in the stools. It can aggravate postural hypotension.

In persistent diabetic diarrhoea, standard anti-diarrhoeals are of some help, albeit incomplete. Loperamide is the first to be tried—codeine phosphate in high doses may be sedative and addictive. Somatostatin is of value if there is a secretory component.

CONSTIPATION

Constipation is a very common problem throughout the normal population. It also is found in diabetics. It may well be related to the diet, although modern dietetic techniques have encouraged the use of unrefined and therefore high-fibre foods. There may well be a change in the innervation of the gut which reveals itself by the development of constipation. If it is a new symptom it will need investigating, particularly in the older patient to exclude an obstructing lesion such as a carcinoma. A bulking agent with ispaghula combined with a stool softening agent such as magnesium hydroxide (contraindicated in renal failure) or dioctyl are crucial to getting a soft stool. If there is still a problem with defecation then a muscle stimulant such as senna may be used—up to a maximum of, say, twice a week, so as to reduce the tendency for tolerance, and mucosal damage from the stimulant laxative.

BILIARY TRACT

There may well be an increase in gall stones in diabetics. One would expect this, particularly in the NIDDM patients who tend to be overweight. Recent studies suggest that when account is taken of body weight there is no increased incidence, although there may be some delayed gall bladder emptying as part of an autonomic neuropathy.

It is worth noting, however, that acute cholecystitis in diabetics carries a significantly increased morbidity and mortality. Early referral to hospital, with early blood cultures to obtain an organism, and broad spectrum, powerful antibiotics are required. Good ultrasound is needed at an early stage with a view to early endoscopic intervention (ERCP) if it is felt that there may be a stone in the common bile duct.

LIVER

The association between the liver and diabetes is strong, and two-way. Diabetes may affect the liver, the liver may affect the diabetes, and there may also be a common factor connecting the two.

HEPATIC DYSFUNCTION CAUSED BY DIABETES

By far the commonest hepatic complication of diabetes is a fatty liver. This is strongly associated with obesity, therefore with Type II diabetes. Fat droplets are found in a substantial proportion of the hepatocytes, displacing the nucleus, with an associated mild inflammatory infiltrate. Liver function tests are usually mildly disturbed, with the alkaline phosphatase elevated 20 to 50%, and the transaminases at the upper end of normal or just above. There is no jaundice. An ultrasound will often show a rather bright reflective pattern diffusely throughout the liver. It does not cause any disease, although often causes anxiety because of the changes in liver function—however, an anxiety that seldom seems to lead to a serious reduction in weight despite advice given. A reduction in ingestion of fat and a genuine weight loss will resolve this. It is probable that this is aggravated by alcohol which can also cause a fatty liver by a different mechanism, and excess alcohol imbibing is in the differential diagnosis.

LIVER DISEASE DUE TO DIABETES

At one stage it was felt that viral hepatitis (particularly B and non-A, non-B) was increased due to contamination of needles. Now that individuals have their own equipment with disposable needles this is not a problem.

Oral hypoglycaemic drugs may induce liver enzymes. Sulphonyl ureas can lead to a number of side effects, one of which is a cholestatic jaundice.

LIVER DISEASE LINKED WITH DIABETES

Haemochromatosis is a congenital abnormality of iron absorption in which excess iron is absorbed and is deposited in a number of organs in the body. In particular the pancreas, gonads and liver may be involved. Through damage by excess iron in the pancreas diabetes may follow and excess iron in the liver may lead to progressive hepatic deterioration and ultimately cirrhosis. Very high serum iron levels are found.

LIVER DISEASE CAUSING A DIABETIC-LIKE PROBLEM

Liver disease, particularly if severe and chronic, may lead to carbohydrate intolerance, with a reduced gluconeogenesis, so that hypoglycaemia may follow exercise in the fasting state. Impaired glycogenolysis can also result from chronic liver disease, leading to temporary hyperglycaemia after a meal. Care needs to be taken in assessing whether the individual has diabetes, so as to decide whether any treatment is necessary—other than small, regular meals.

ACUTE PROBLEMS WITH DIABETIC KETOACIDOSIS

Acute diabetic ketoacidosis not uncommonly leads to a picture of an acute abdomen, with tense, board-like rigidity, severe abdominal pain, tachycardia, and of course dehydration and hyperglycaemia. It is all too easy for the inexperienced doctor to think that the abdominal crisis has triggered the ketoacidosis. A very important rule is *never* to operate on a supposed acute abdomen while the patient's diabetes is out of control with severe hyperglycaemia and ketoacidosis, unless there is cast iron evidence of an intra-abdominal catastrophe, such as a perforation. Even so it is better to wait until rehydration has taken place, electrolytes are in balance, the blood sugar coming down and the abdomen can be reassessed. Such standard treatment of diabetic ketoacidosis has resolved many an apparent acute abdomen—be conservative!

CONCLUSION

Disordered function of the gastrointestinal tract is very common in the general population and therefore diabetics. However, some of the diabetic complications can be particularly troublesome, our understanding of them is incomplete, and management not always satisfactory. Careful assessment with the history and detailed investigation, can often give a basis upon which rational therapy can be employed.

REFERENCES

1 Jones R, Lydeard S. Dyspepsia in the community: a follow up study. *Br J Clin Pract* 1992; **46**: 95–7.
2 Janatuinen E, Pikkarainen P, Laakso M, Pyorala K. Gastrointestinal symptoms in middle-aged diabetic patients. *Scan J Gastroenterol* 1993; **28**: 427–32.
3 Borgstrom P, Olsson R, Sundkvist G *et al*. Pharyngeal and oesophageal function in patients with diabetes mellitus and swallowing complaints. *Br J Radiol* 1988; **61**: 817–21.
4 Falchuk KR, Conlin D. The intestinal and liver complications of diabetes mellitus. *Adv Int Med* 1993; **38**: 269–86.
5 Kassander P. Asymptomatic gastric retention in diabetics (gastroparesis diabeticorum). *Ann Intern Med* 1958; **48**: 797–804.
6 Colin-Jones DG *et al*. Management of dyspepsia: report of a working party. *Lancet* 1988; **1**: 576–9.
7 Drenth JPH, Engels LGJB. Diabetic gastroparesis. *Drugs* 1992; **44**(4): 538–53.
8 Horowitz M, Dent J. Disordered gastric emptying: mechanical basis, assessment and treatment. *Bailliere's Clinical Gastroenterology* 1991; **5**: 371–407.
9 Horowitz M, Maddox A, Harding PE, Maddern GJ, Chatterton BE *et al*. Effect of cisapride on gastric and esophageal emptying in insulin-dependent diabetes mellitus. *Gastroenterology* 1987; **92**: 1899–1907.
10 Malagelada JR. Diabetic gastroparesis in perspective. *Gastroenterology* 1994; **107**: 581–3.
11 Farthing MJG. Bacterial overgrowth of the small intestine. In: Misiewicz JJ,

Pounder RE, Venables CW (eds), *Diseases of the Gut and Pancreas*. Oxford: Blackwell, 1987.

12 Unsworth DJ, Brown DL. Serological screening suggests that adult coeliac disease is underdiagnosed in the U.K. and increases the incidence by up to 12%. *Gut* 1994; **35**: 61–4.

13 Bilous RW. Diabetic autonomic neuropathy. *BMJ* 1990; **301**: 565–7.

14 Valdovinos MA, Camilleri M, Zimmerman BR. Chronic diarrhoea in diabetes mellitus: mechanisms and an approach to diagnosis and treatment. *Mayo Clin Proc* 1993; **68**: 691–702.

15 Ogbonnaya KI, Arem R. Diabetic diarrhoea. *Arch Intern Med* 1990; **150**: 262–7.

16 Mourad FH, Gorard D, Thillainayagam AV, Colin-Jones DG, Farthing MJG. Effective treatment of diabetic diarrhoea with somatostatin analogue, octreotide. *Gut* 1992; **33**: 1578–80.

6

Diabetic Neuropathy

A. MACLEOD and P. SÖNKSEN*

Royal Shrewsbury Hospital, Shrewsbury and *Department of Endocrinology and
Chemical Pathology, St Thomas' Hospital, London

HISTORICAL PERSPECTIVE

Since the nineteenth century, it has been recognized that diabetes mellitus
affects the nervous system. Marchal de Calvi is reputed to be the first to
comment in writing, in 1864, that peripheral neuropathy might result from
diabetes[1]. Ogle, in 1866, also described cases 'of diabetes in which ... dis-
turbances of the nervous system appear to stand in the relation of consequence or result of the diabetic state'[2]. The abnormalities that Ogle
described, however, were of the brain and spinal cord, rather than the
peripheral nerves. Before their hypotheses, it had in fact been assumed
that damage to the nervous system was responsible for, rather than a consequence of, the diabetic state, encouraged by the experiments of Claude
Bernard on the fourth ventricle of the brain where destructive lesions
resulted in hyperglycaemia[3].

Jendrassik published a paper on the usefulness of the tendon reflex
response in assessing neuropathy, and also a method for its accentuation
(now called 'reinforcement' or the 'Jendrassik manoeuvre') in 1883[4]. One
year later, Bouchard reported that the patellar tendon reflex response was
absent in some patients with diabetes, probably, he thought, as a result of
neuropathic damage. Of 66 diabetic patients that he examined, 19 had
absent patellar tendon reflexes. Those without reflexes tended to have a
poor prognosis; six out of 19 died within 3 years, compared with two out
of 47 patients with reflexes[5]. Williamson surveyed the subject in 1897 and

Diabetic Complications. Edited by K. M. Shaw
© 1996 John Wiley & Sons Ltd

found that the knee-jerks were absent in about 50% of his cases in Manchester, a high figure which he considered to be due to the severity of the patients' disease[6]. Six years later he reported the absence of both the Tendo-Achilles jerk and vibration sense in the feet using the tuning fork in patients with diabetes[7].

A classic and detailed description of the symptoms of diabetic polyneuropathy was subsequently provided by the Guy's Hospital physician, Pavy, in 1885[8]. He described the symptoms as 'of darting or lightning pains... Or there may be hyperaesthesia, so that a mere pinching up of the skin gives rise to great pain ... and I have noticed that these pains are generally worse at night'. He also stated that some patients could not 'feel properly in their legs', and that these features might be accompanied by the loss of the patellar tendon reflex. This phenomenon he regarded 'as simply an issue of the toxic action of the sugar contaminating the system upon the nerves'. He was also fully aware of the distressing consequences of neuropathy: the 'perforating sore ... leading into the joint of a toe or to denuded bone.... There is usually a prolonged history of diabetic neuritis'.

A copy of a contemporary photograph of Pavy who, despite being a pupil of Claude Bernard, spent most of his research effort trying to disprove Bernard's still valid hypothesis of generation of glucose by the liver, is shown in Figure 6.1.

Evidence that autonomic nerve function might be affected in diabetes mellitus was also provided in the second half of the nineteenth century. Pavy reported on the involvement of the vasomotor system, and also that localized areas of abnormal sweating might become apparent. Like Ogle, he also reported the association of impotence and diabetes in 1904[9].

Most of the clinical features of neuropathy in diabetes were recognized before the discovery and treatment of patients with insulin in 1923. These descriptions were almost certainly from patients with non-insulin-dependent diabetes, who had managed to survive the 5 years or so now thought to be necessary for the irreversible features of diabetic nerve damage to become clinically detectable.

One of the first descriptions of the use of electrophysiological techniques in the assessment of diabetic neuropathy was provided by Buzzard in 1890[10]. He applied induced current to the lower limbs of a diabetic patient with bilateral foot drop and found the motor response to be impaired. Reliable and repeatable measurement of nerve conduction and methods of quantifying sensation in the feet of patients with diabetes were not developed until the 1950s.

It was left to Rundles, in 1945[11], to provide what would still be considered a comprehensive description of the features of diabetic autonomic

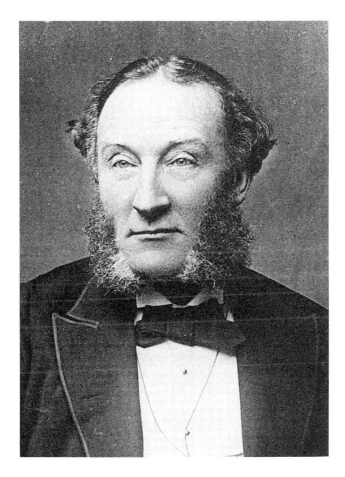

Figure 6.1. F.W. Pavy, the Guy's Hospital physician who first described the symptoms of diabetic polyneuropathy in 1885. (Courtesy of Andrew Basta, UMDS Library Services)

neuropathy. He described abnormalities of temperature regulation, pupillary function, postural hypotension, vasomotor control, intestinal and bladder function, and also reiterated the problem of impotence in the male. During the second half of the twentieth century the protean manifestations of diabetic autonomic neuropathy have been recognized, and attempts made to classify and define the different syndromes of nerve damage seen in patients with diabetes.

CLASSIFICATION OF DIABETIC NEUROPATHIES

Diabetes may affect both the central and peripheral nerves. Involvement of the central nervous system may be transient; coma, convulsions or even focal neurological signs may be associated with a hypoglycaemic attack, and focal epilepsy is a rare but well-recognized accompaniment of the hyperglycaemic hyperosmolar state. Cerebrovascular accidents are four times as common in the diabetic as opposed to the non-diabetic population, due to the increased incidence of macrovascular disease. The term 'diabetic neuropathy', however, is usually taken to encompass the spectrum of damage to the peripheral nerves that is seen in diabetes. A working classification of diabetic neuropathies, adapted from Thomas and Eliasson[12], is given in Table 6.1.

ACUTE SENSORIMOTOR NEUROPATHY

Hyperglycaemia is known to affect peripheral nerve function after as little time as a few hours. This effect has been demonstrated in studies on animals and in studies in human subjects with or even without diabetes[13]. Patients with newly diagnosed diabetes may have symptoms typical of neuropathy, and are known to have slowed nerve conduction velocity both of which usually recover rapidly with treatment[14,15]. This acute neuropathy may therefore occur with any short period of hyperglycaemia, and has a good prognosis provided the diabetes is satisfactorily controlled. Whether the same biochemical process is responsible for the more irreversible changes seen in chronic neuropathy is not known. Possible mechanisms are discussed below.

Table 6.1. A simple classification of diabetic neuropathies

Sensorimotor neuropathy
- Acute
- Chronic

Autonomic neuropathy

Mononeuropathy
- Spontaneous
- Entrapment
- External pressure palsies

Proximal motor neuropathy

CHRONIC SENSORIMOTOR NEUROPATHY

DEFINITION AND PREVALENCE

Despite much discussion there is no universally agreed definition of diabetic sensorimotor neuropathy. The problem is in the variety of ways that peripheral nerve function can be assessed. The more sensitive tests, such as nerve conduction velocity, or the measurement of the compound nerve action potential, may pick up an abnormality in up to 80% of the diabetic population. The relevance of such abnormalities to the life of the patient is difficult to interpret at present, and may sometimes be reversible, as stated above. Most diabetologists prefer to stick to a definition that is based upon definite abnormalities detected on clinical examination, while recognizing that this may be at a relatively late stage in the pathological process. Some authorities prefer to use a summation score of clinical signs (NDS or Neurological Disability Score) to exclude patients with minor deficits that may still be in the normal range[16,17]. Such a system is described below and given in Table 6.2. Neuropathic symptoms may not reflect the degree of damage to the nerve, and are best excluded from the basic definition in our opinion. Patients may, therefore, have chronic sensorimotor neuropathy 'with or without symptoms'.

It must be remembered that there is as yet no specific test for diabetic neuropathy. To be confident that the neuropathy is due to the diabetes alone, the clinician must first exclude other causes of peripheral sensorimotor neuropathy. A list of other possibilities is given in Table 6.3. It goes

Table 6.2. A scoring system for the signs of diabetic peripheral neuropathy*

NEUROPATHY EXAMINATION

SENSATION

	RIGHT		LEFT	
	NORMAL	ABNORMAL	NORMAL	ABNORMAL
Pain (pin prick)	0	1	0	1
Vibration (tuning fork)	0	1	0	1
Temperature (cold metal)	0	1	0	1

ACHILLES REFLEX

RIGHT			LEFT		
PRESENT	REINFORCE ONLY	ABSENT	PRESENT	REINFORCE ONLY	ABSENT
0	1	2	0	1	2

NEUROPATHY SCORE = [____] (0 to 10)

* Adapted from Young *et al*[18]

Table 6.3. Differential diagnosis of diabetic peripheral neuropathy

Toxic
- Uraemia
- Industrial and environmental
  - Acrylamide
  - Arsenic
  - Lead
  - Mercury
  - Thallium
  - Triorthocresyl phosphate
- Drug induced
  - Isoniazid
  - Nitrofurantoin
  - Vincristine
  - Thalidomide

Deficiency neuropathies
- Beri beri
- Alcoholic neuropathy
- Pernicious anaemia
- Pyridoxine deficiency
- Pantothenic acid deficiency
- Vitamin E deficiency

Infiltrative and Inflammatory
- Amyloidosis
- Leprosy
- Acute idiopathic inflammatory neuropathy (Guillain-Barré)
- Chronic idiopathic inflammatory neuropathy
- Acquired immunodeficiency syndrome
- Sarcoidosis

Endocrine
- Myxoedema
- Acromegaly

Neoplastic

Paraproteinaemia

Genetic
- Porphyria
- Peroneal muscular atrophy
- Other hereditary neuropathies

without saying that if the clinical course of any patient who has been diagnosed as having diabetic neuropathy begins to show atypical features, then there should be a thorough examination to search for other causes. Uraemia is particularly important as it may exacerbate pre-existing diabetic neuropathy in patients on renal support regimens and therefore be overlooked; it then represents an indication for urgent renal transplantation. Myxoedema and B_{12} deficiency are associated with diabetes in the polyendocrine autoimmune syndrome.

A number of studies have examined the prevalence of clinically defined peripheral neuropathy in the diabetic population. One large study of 6487 patients examined with a simple clinical scoring system in 119 hospital diabetes centres in the United Kingdom has revealed an overall prevalence of neuropathy of 28.5%[18]. The prevalence of neuropathy increased markedly with age, and with duration of diabetes; 44.2% of 70 to 79-year-olds were affected, and 36.8% after more than 10 years of known diabetes. Population-derived studies suggest that the prevalence of neuropathy may be even higher in the community, perhaps due to the increase in the average age of those being treated in the community versus the hospital clinic population[19]. As we have said, the prevalence of patients with abnormalities of nerve function increases still further when sensitive tests such as measurement of sural sensory nerve conduction velocity are used.

CLINICAL FEATURES

Although motor nerves are clearly affected, diabetic peripheral neuropathy is predominantly sensory, and the distribution is usually symmetrical. The condition first affects the most distal parts of the longest nerves in the body (i.e. the toes and soles of the feet). The hands are only clinically affected with severe and longstanding neuropathy. In the most severe cases, it may be possible to detect numbness over the mid-sternal area, due to involvement of the ends of the intercostal nerves[12].

Symptoms

Neuropathic symptoms consist of the following:

- Pain, which may be sharp, stabbing or burning, particularly on the soles of the feet or shins

- Skin tenderness (hyperpathia or hyperaesthesia)

- Pins and needles (paraesthesia) and a positive feeling of numbness.

These symptoms may be excruciating and unremitting, and tend to be exacerbated at night, keeping the patient awake. There is, however, little correlation between the degree of nerve damage and the presence of symptoms. Patients with no complaints whatsoever may be found on examination to have completely anaesthetic feet: a particularly dangerous situation. In a study of patients in the diabetic clinic at St Thomas'

Hospital, London, approximately 50% of patients with clinical evidence of neuropathy (on examination) were asymptomatic as far as the feet were concerned[20].

Clinical Signs

Decreased vibration sense and absent ankle jerks are the earliest and most useful clinical signs of diabetic neuropathy, followed by muscular weakness and wasting when the condition is severe. As diabetes produces a symmetrical distal neuropathy, it is best to test the extremes of both feet, e.g. the hallux.

The scoring system described in Table 6.2 takes 2 to 3 minutes to carry out and uses methods that are part of routine medical training. The only instruments necessary are a tendon hammer, a disposable pin, and a 128 Hz tuning fork. The latter can be used as the cold metal implement, and can be compared with the examiner's index finger across the dorsum of the hallux or distal foot. The score can be used to categorize neuropathy as follows:

0–2: No neuropathy
3–5: Mild neuropathy
6–8: Moderate neuropathy
9,10: Severe neuropathy

This score can then be used to select patients at risk of foot problems for more intensive treatment such as food education programmes and regular visits to the chiropodist. During the examination the feet can be carefully inspected for the presence of foot problems, and pulses felt to detect peripheral vascular disease.

ADDITIONAL TESTS

In addition to the neurological pin, cotton wool swab, and conventional tuning fork other tests have been developed to increase the accuracy of diagnosis, and provide a quantifiable means of assessing sensory nerve function that can be compared more easily between observers.

Rydel Seiffer Tuning Fork

A simple improvement is the modification of the conventional tuning fork, devised by Rydel and Seiffer, by applying calibrated weights to the prongs and therefore allowing some quantification of this sensory test[21]. Their graduated tuning fork has recently been reassessed and found to be an inexpensive improvement on the conventional fork for the assessment of diabetic neuropathy by Liniger and colleagues[22].

Monofilaments

An equally simple method of measuring cutaneous sensation is the application of monofilaments to the skin to assess pressure sensation. Semmes and Weinstein have modified Von Frey hairs into a set of nylon monofilaments[23]. Buckling of the filament above a certain threshold allows a relatively constant application of pressure to a small area of skin, which can be altered by using a number of filaments of differing circumference. In this way a semiquantitative and repeatable means of testing pressure sensation may be obtained which can detect the difference between, for instance, patients with clinical evidence of neuropathy but with or without a history of foot ulceration[24].

The Biothesiometer, Neurothesiometer

The Biothesiometer (Biomedical Instrument Co., Newbury, Ohio, USA) has been available for clinical use since the early 1950s, and has more recently been updated as the battery powered Neurothesiometer (Scientific Laboratory Supplies Ltd, Nottingham, UK)[25]. The design is simple and robust. A hand-held device containing a vibrating polyethylene probe is placed against the skin. The vibrating frequency of 100–120 Hz is sufficient to stimulate mainly the Pacinian corpuscles in the skin. Varying the voltage alters the amplitude of vibration. The amplitude is increased until the subject states that he or she can feel the vibration: this is the 'Vibration Perception Threshold' or VPT. The pressure applied with the probe is recommended to approximate to the weight of the instrument; increasing the pressure decreases the amplitude of vibration and has been found to alter the vibration threshold[26]. As with virtually all tests of peripheral nerve function skin temperature is important and the feet should be warm[27].

Normal ranges for different ages are available for the Biothesiometer[28,80]. Most clinicians use the thumb pulp, the bony prominence of the medial malleolus or just the great toe pulp as sites of measurement. A useful property of the range is that the log VPT is linearly related with age. Given the coefficients, therefore, the reading can easily be corrected for age and translated into standard deviations from the mean of normal with a programmable calculator[29].

The VPT therefore provides a quantitative estimate of neuropathy. Boulton has found that the development of foot problems usually occurs in patients with a VPT of at least 35 volts as measured at the great toe;

these patients can therefore be targeted for enhanced foot care pro-grammes[30].

More sophisticated devices for the measurement of vibration threshold have more recently been produced. For example the Vibrameter (Somedic, Sweden) incorporates an optical device at the vibrating head which directly measures the amplitude of vibration regardless of the voltage delivered to the instrument, and also has a visual indicator of the pressure applied at the tip. In our view the benefit of this sophistication is out-weighed by the ease of use of the simpler (and cheaper) Biothesiometer or Neurothesiometer for the purposes of the clinic. These tests of cutaneous vibration and pressure sense are thought to investigate the function of large, fast, myelinated afferent nerve fibres[31].

The Neurometer

The Neurometer (Minimed Technologies, Sylmar, Calif., USA) is a battery operated device that can provide a constant current stimulus as a sine wave of up to 10 mA. The output of the current generator is maintained continuously by a feedback circuit during the procedure, so that altera-tions in skin resistance are automatically accommodated. Three different frequencies are possible: 5 Hz, 250 Hz, and 2 kHz.

The device provides good discrimination between neuropathic and non-neuropathic diabetic patients; high frequencies correlate best with tests of large fibre function, and low frequencies with tests of small fibre function[32,33]. There is no published evidence, however, to suggest that the device is superior to the Biothesiometer for the assessment of diabetic neuropathy.

Measurement of Temperature Sensation

Cutaneous sensations of cold (and pricking pain) are thought to be trans-mitted by small myelinated fibres, and sensations of warmth (and aching, deep pain) by unmyelinated fibres[31]. Quantification of temperature sense required the development of a device that could produce a rapid and varied but predictable change in temperature. Such properties were achieved by the development of the Marstock apparatus, which utilizes Peltier elements that produce a negative or positive change in temperature depending on the direction and magnitude of applied electrical current[34]. Computerized, forced-choice automation systems have considerably improved precision[35,36], but there is still considerable variability on repeated testing[37]. These tests are lengthy and require a considerable amount of concentration from the patient. They are therefore not suitable for routine clinical use and remain useful only for research.

Electrophysiological Assessment of Nerve Function

The technique of measurement of nerve conduction is well established and is now routinely used in neurology for the diagnosis and assessment of peripheral neuropathy. The relevant nerve is stimulated by a brief pulse of electrical current, and the response recorded either by surface or needle electrodes, over the innervated muscle to measure the compound muscle action potential (CMAP) or 'M-wave' in the case of the motor nerve, or over the nerve itself to measure the sensory nerve action potential (SNAP) in the case of the sensory nerve. The response of the latter is some 100 times smaller than the CMAP, and therefore a digital averager is used with multiple stimulation in order to define the response with enough accuracy. To measure conduction velocity the nerve is stimulated at two sites, as far apart as possible, and the distance between the sites is divided by the different response times to derive the velocity. This is particularly important for the CMAP as this response includes a significant delay due to neuromuscular transmission.

The easiest and most repeatable method of calculating the response takes the beginning of the action potential as the relevant time point, hence this measurement looks at the fastest conducting fibres only. Measurement of the amplitude of the response gives some indication of the total number of fibres stimulated, which is more accurately assessed by the area under the response. This may be difficult to measure in a damaged nerve, and varies dramatically according to placement of electrodes, etc.

Nerve conduction velocity is affected by skin temperature, and deteriorates (like most things) with increasing age[38]. As mentioned above, it can be changed rapidly (over hours) by large alterations in blood glucose[13].

Another technique has been developed to examine the speed of conduction of the motor nerves in the upper rather than the lower part of the limb, termed the 'F-wave response'[39-41]. Depolarizing the motor fibres with the electrical stimulus produces an antidromic (opposite to the usual physiological direction of travel) as well as an orthodromic nerve impulse. This travels up to the anterior horn cell, and after a delay of about 1 ms another impulse curiously travels orthodromically down the nerve fibre, and can be picked up at the muscle electrode considerably later than the 'M response'. This response reflects a single motor unit, and therefore an estimate of the *average* speed of the fibres can be gained from a number of stimulations[42]. This test might have an advantage in picking up nerve damage at an early stage.

These electrophysiological tests need expertise and experience to perform, and take many minutes if not hours. Unlike the more complex tests of sensation, however, they are objective, require only relaxation on behalf of the patient, and are less variable in day-to-day testing[37]. They may pick up an abnormality at an earlier stage. At present neuroelectrophysiological assessment is only relevant to atypical cases, or as a measure of response in research trials. If a treatment were to become available that could affect neuropathy at an early stage, it might become an important part of clinical routine.

AETIOLOGY

The development of diabetic neuropathy is known to be associated with increasing duration of diabetes, and with poor blood glucose control[43]. Clinical trials that assess the benefit of improved blood glucose control in patients with insulin-dependent diabetes have shown that improved control decreases both the incidence and the progression of neuropathy[44]. A number of hypotheses exist to explain how the cumulative exposure to high glucose levels may predispose to the development of neuropathy. No clear genetic influences (e.g. HLA type) have yet been proven to be relevant to the selection of those who develop neuropathy.

The Aldose Reductase Hypothesis

The aldose reductase hypothesis has been invoked for many years to explain some of the chronic complications of diabetes mellitus. The hypothesis proposes that a minor biochemical pathway becomes overactive in diabetes and brings about tissue damage. It has remained a viable hypothesis for a number of years, particularly because the pathway has been shown to be active in the relevant tissues and cells concerned with diabetic complications, is further activated in diabetic states, and is known to produce functional abnormalities in many animal models of diabetes[45]. Its role in the generation of diabetic complications in the human, however, is still contentious and unclear.

Aldose reductase is the rate-limiting enzyme of the sorbitol or polyol pathway, whereby glucose is converted to sorbitol and then to fructose via the enzyme sorbitol dehydrogenase. Aldose reductase is activated by high concentrations of glucose, thus markedly increasing the flux through the pathway in diabetes[46]. The hypothesis is that this increased flux results in the depletion of essential co-factors in the cell, thereby causing acute and then chronic malfunction of the nerve. Inhibitors of aldose reductase are now available; these can reverse or prevent most acute changes seen in animal models of diabetic neuropathy[47-49]. They are now being used in clinical studies to investigate the role of the sorbitol pathway and any therapeutic implications. To date they have been shown to increase nerve conduction velocity in patients with diabetic neuropathy[50-52]; we await further studies to assess whether such changes translate into real clinical benefit with continued use.

Hypoxia

Studies of nerves in animal models of diabetes and in patients with diabetic neuropathy have demonstrated endoneurial hypoxia, which may be due to abnormalities in the microvascular supply to the nerve[53,54]. Tissue hypoxia is known to result in abnormal nerve function, but it remains to be proven whether this is true for diabetic neuropathy[55]. This hypothesis is attractive as it is paralleled by the known effects of diabetes on the microvascular supply of the retina; such changes could of course be brought about by endothelial cell damage via the polyol pathway[56].

Non-enzymatic Glycosylation

Non-enzymatic glycosylation of structural proteins has been put forward as an aetiological factor in the development of diabetic retinopathy and nephropathy. So far it has little support as a cause of the development of neuropathy.

TREATMENT OF DIABETIC PERIPHERAL NEUROPATHY

Prevention of Neuropathy

Clinical trials, now including the large DCCT (Diabetes Control and Complications Trial) from the United States[44] have revealed clear benefits of improved blood glucose control on diabetic neuropathy in patients with insulin-dependent diabetes. Prevention or amelioration of nerve damage is therefore one of many reasons to support our (i.e. patient + health care worker) efforts in the diabetic clinic to achieve near-normal control for these patients. It is tempting to extrapolate these findings to patients with non-insulin-dependent diabetes; the same benefits may not apply here in view of the duration of diabetes at diagnosis and the older average age of the patients (and therefore the potential of recovery of nerve damage).

Prevention of Foot Damage

Measures to prevent damage to the feet in patients with neuropathy are an essential part of diabetic care (see Chapter 7). As neuropathy may be symptomless, screening is essential to be able to focus on those who are most at risk.

Treatment of Symptoms

The pain of diabetic neuropathy can be extremely distressing and unremitting, often lasting throughout the night. The pain usually improves with time[57], especially when associated with recently improved blood glucose control, and it is worth pointing this out to the patient who may have assumed that its course is endless. It does not usually respond to conventional analgesia. If there is a significant degree of hyperaesthesia it is worth trying contact dressings such as 'Opsite' particularly over the hypersensitive areas such as the shin or dorsum of the foot[58]. Another topical treatment that has been shown to be effective in double-blind trials is the application of capsaicin cream[81].

The tricyclic antidepressants, e.g. amitriptyline or imipramine have a specific effect on the neuropathic symptoms of diabetic neuropathy. They may provide dramatic relief of symptoms within 48 hours, well before their antidepressant effect, and are as effective in patients with or without clinically defined depression[59]: their mode of action is therefore thought to be via a different route. Amitriptyline, in a single dose of 25 mg at bedtime and increasing to 75 mg or even 100 mg if necessary, is usually effective throughout the day, and also has a nocturnal sedative effect which is particularly useful when the painful symptoms have nocturnal exacerbation, as is often the case. Side effects include sedation persisting until the next day, a dry mouth, urinary retention and postural hypotension, which is especially a problem in patients with significant autonomic neuropathy. For those patients who receive benefit from amitriptyline but cannot tolerate the sedative side effects, imipramine or desipramine, a relatively specific blocker of noradrenaline re-uptake, have been shown to be equally effective, at a similar dose. Similar drugs with less anticholinergic side effects, e.g. the inhibitor of serotonin re-uptake, fluoxetine, or the serotonin antagonist mianserin, have disappointingly little effect on symptoms[59,60]. Paroxetine, at a dose of 40 mg/day has been reported to be more effective than placebo, although less so than imipramine[61]. Other second line drugs for the treatment of symptoms include carbamazepine, at mild to moderate doses, phenytoin or mexilitine, all of which are proven to exert some benefit[62]. All have well-documented side effects which may restrict their action.

If there is little response to these agents, or if there are any other atypical features, a search should be made for other causes of the patient's symptoms.

DIABETIC AUTONOMIC NEUROPATHY

Impaired function of the small unmyelinated nerve fibres involved in the control of the autonomic nervous system is common in diabetes. As many as 40% of patients with diabetes may have an abnormality on testing autonomic nerve function[63]. Only a small percentage, however, have classical symptoms (excluding impotence); these patients usually have minimal or no cardiovascular responses, i.e. severe nerve damage. In diagnosis and management it is important to distinguish between these two features. Patients with *symptomatic* diabetic autonomic neuropathy have been found to have a high cumulative mortality, partly due to associated nephropathy but also due to a higher than expected incidence of sudden death[64]. Subsequent studies have been less pessimistic, but the possibility remains that severely disordered autonomic function in these patients may occasionally result in catastrophe[65].

AETIOLOGY

As in sensorimotor neuropathy, the prevalence of autonomic neuropathy increases with the duration of the disease and with poor control of blood glucose. There is close correlation between tests of peripheral sensory and peripheral autonomic nerve function[66]. As might be expected the two types of clinical neuropathy are often seen in the same patient; most patients with clinically important autonomic neuropathy have evidence of marked sensorimotor involvement. These similarities with peripheral sensorimotor neuropathy have led to the suggestion of the same pathological process being involved, at least in the early stages of nerve damage. There is some evidence of a beneficial effect of aldose reductase inhibition on autonomic function tests (not symptoms) in patients with diabetes[67]. We await further studies to determine whether the polyol pathway is the culprit and whether we have a specific means of treatment.

Symptomatic autonomic neuropathy is particularly rare in non-insulin-dependent diabetes[68]. There is also a curious but well documented association of iritis with this stage of autonomic neuropathy in patients with insulin-dependent diabetes[69]. Antibodies to components of nerve cells and inflammatory cells in nerve biopsies have been found in affected subjects, which has led to the suggestion that early damage to autonomic nerves triggers an autoimmune destructive process that in turn accentuates the progression of autonomic neuropathy in these symptomatic patients[57]. These findings may simply be a response to nerve damage rather than a cause[70].

There may be a genetic predisposition to the development of autonomic neuropathy in diabetes[71].

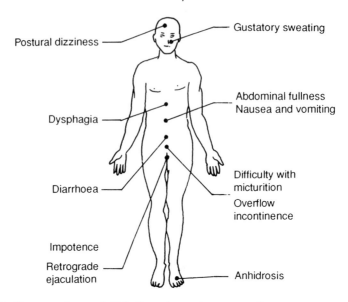

Figure 6.2. The symptoms of diabetic autonomic neuropathy

SYMPTOMS

Numerous symptoms can be ascribed to diabetic autonomic neuropathy
(Figure 6.2). Autonomic neuropathy is a major component of erectile
impotence, which may occur in at least 35% of diabetic adult males[72].
Other clinically important symptoms include dizziness and blackouts due
to postural hypotension, and nausea and vomiting due to gastroparesis,
which may be exacerbated by hyperglycaemia, infections or pregnancy[73].
Absent sweating over the lower half of the body is rarely recognized by
the subject, but increased sweating over the upper half of the trunk and
face may be distressing especially at night. Gustatory sweating, that is
facial sweating when eating, is rare but a particular feature of symptomatic diabetic autonomic neuropathy and may embarrass the
patient[74,75], as may diabetic diarrhoea which usually occurs in bouts of a
few days.

CLINICAL SIGNS

Signs include dry skin due to absence of sweating, particularly over the
feet and shins, postural hypotension, tachycardia with no sinus arrythmia,
and small pupils. Twenty-four-hour ambulatory monitoring of blood
pressure may reveal a paradoxical pattern of highest pressure overnight
and lowest in the morning[76].

DIAGNOSIS

There is a vast array of tests described for the diagnosis of autonomic dysfunction. Ewing has proposed a 'battery' of five simple non-invasive tests: the heart rate response to the Valsalva manoeuvre; the heart rate response to standing up; the heart rate response to deep breathing; the blood pressure response to standing up; and the blood pressure response to sustained handgrip[77].

Most clinical situations are resolved in our experience by the use of only two of these tests.

Measurement of the blood pressure response to standing (systolic drop of >20 mmHg on standing, best measured after 2 minutes) helps to assess whether postural symptoms are due to autonomic neuropathy.

The heart rate response to deep breathing (the 'E:I ratio') provides a quick, easy and more sensitive test of autonomic dysfunction. While resting on a couch and connected to an ECG machine, the subject is asked to take a single maximal deep breath, lasting about 5 seconds in, 5 seconds out. The shortest R–R interval (during inspiration) and the longest (expiration) are measured on the paper and the expired to inspired ('E:I') ratio calculated. Normal values for an age-related range have been published[78].

TREATMENT

General Measures

Patients with autonomic neuropathy are unable to adapt rapidly to changes in intravascular volume or to changes in posture. They therefore need special care during anaesthesia and in the perioperative period.

Postural Hypotension

Postural hypotension may be helped by simple measures such as avoiding any dehydration, slow resumption of the upright posture, elevation of the head of the bed to try to maintain plasma volume at night, and support stockings. A check for medications that exacerbate postural hypotension must be made. Fludrocortisone is the mainstay of treatment, and doses of 0.1 to 0.4 mg daily may be necessary. The main side effects are supine hypertension, hypokalaemia and oedema. Other agents that have some effect are the alpha adrenergic agonist midodrine, a retiring dose of desmopressin, and octreotide[79].

Abnormal Sweating, Gastroparesis, Diarrhoea

Anticholinergics (e.g. propantheline bromide or poldine methylsulphate) may help excessive or gustatory sweating. Exacerbation of postural hypotension or urinary retention may restrict their use.

The nausea and vomiting of diabetic gastroparesis may be exacerbated by intercurrent illness which must be vigorously treated. Metoclopramide, domperidone, and cisapride are drugs of choice (suppositories may be effective if the patient is vomiting).

One or two days of oral tetracycline (250 mg twice daily) may control diabetic diarrhoea. The mechanism is obscure but may be via the reduction of bacterial overgrowth. Antidiarrhoeal agents such as codeine phosphate, or loperamide may help.

DIABETIC MONONEUROPATHIES

Spontaneous neuropathies, external pressure palsies and entrapment neuropathies are all more common in diabetic patients. This increased frequency is thought to be due to the vulnerability of an already compromised peripheral nervous system. Spontaneous neuropathy is of rapid onset, and there is presumably a vascular component in its aetiology, although there is no proof.

SPONTANEOUS NEUROPATHY

Of the spontaneous neuropathies that are related to diabetes, the cranial nerves, particularly the third but also the fourth, sixth and seventh are most often involved. The onset is sudden and may be accompanied by pain. With a third nerve palsy due to diabetes the pupil is usually spared, possibly because of a selective lesion due to vascular occlusion (Figure 6.3). The main differential diagnosis is an aneurysm in the carotid siphon. If due to diabetes the prognosis is good; most patients recover after a period of weeks to months, and can be reassured. No specific treatment is necessary.

EXTERNAL PRESSURE PALSIES

In the limbs, other nerve lesions most often occur at sites of external pressure, for example the radial, ulnar and peroneal nerves. Foot drop can occur after a minor insult such as crossing the legs during air travel. Another example of mononeuropathy is that of cranial nerve involvement in malignant otitis externa. Here chronic infection with *Pseudomonas* involves the adjacent cranial nerve and gives rise to the picture seen in

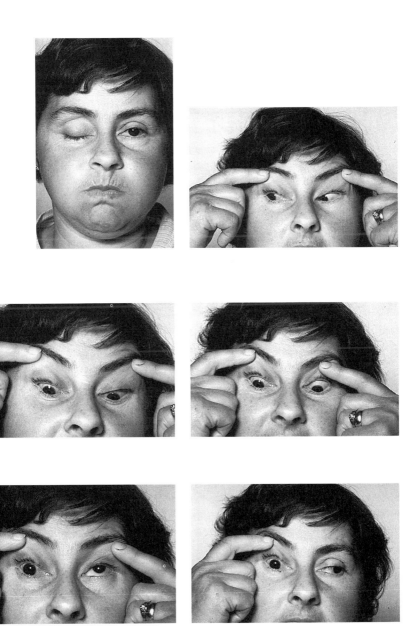

Figure 6.3. Spontaneous third nerve palsy presenting with ptosis

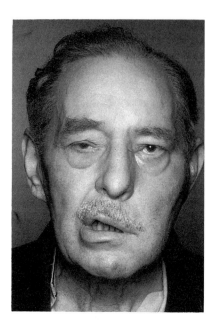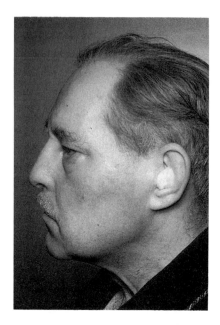

Figure 6.4. Malignant otitis externa presenting as sixth and seventh nerve palsies and a discharging ear

Figure 6.4. Quinolone antibiotics have dramatically improved the prognosis in this previously universally fatal condition.

ENTRAPMENT NEUROPATHIES

Median carpal tunnel syndrome (usually bilateral) may occur in up to 10% of patients in the diabetic clinic. Diagnosis may be difficult in diabetic patients with severe neuropathy involving the hands, where comparison of median and ulnar motor and sensory nerve conduction, or segmental median nerve conduction measurements are necessary[82]. Treatment is by surgical decompression. Entrapment of the lateral cutaneous nerve of the thigh (meralgia paraesthetica) causing pain and paraesthesiae over the lateral aspect of the thigh is also more common in diabetics.

PROXIMAL MOTOR NEUROPATHY (DIABETIC AMYOTROPHY)

Proximal motor neuropathy presents with severe pain, usually asymmetric, paraesthesiae, hyperpathia in the upper legs, and weakness and muscle wasting, especially of the quadriceps[83]. Skin tenderness over the anterior aspect of the thighs and weakness of hip flexion in one or both legs are common clinical signs. Cases of weight loss and weakness without pain have been described[84]. Knee jerks may be absent in the affected side(s). The condition is now known to involve the lower motor neurones of the lumbosacral plexus. It mainly affects middle-aged and elderly patients, and is usually associated with a period of very poor blood glucose control and sometimes with marked weight loss. Diagnosis must exclude other lesions of the sacral plexus, such as lower abdominal malignancy and lumbar disc disease. Amitriptyline can sometimes make a dramatic difference to the pain, which may be excruciating. Insulin may be necessary to achieve good control of blood glucose. The pain and weakness usually improve over weeks or months.

REFERENCES

1 Marchal de Calvi. *Récherches sur les accidents diabetiques*. Paris: P. Asselin, 1864.
2 Ogle JW. On disease of the brain as a result of diabetes mellitus. *St George's Hosp Rep* 1866; **1**: 157–88.
3 Bernard C, Frère. Des troubles nerveux observes chez les diabetiques. *Arch de Neurol*. 1883; **4**: 336.
4 Jendrassik E. Beitrage zur Lehre von den Sehnenreflexen. *Deutsches Archiv für Klinische Medizin* 1883; **33**: 177–99.
5 Bouchard. Sur la perte des reflexes tendineux dans le diabete sucre. *Le Progrès Médicale* 1884: 819.
6 Williamson RT. Note on the Tendo-Achilles jerk and other reflexes in diabetes mellitus. *Rev Neurol Psychiat* 1903; **1**: 667.
7 Williamson RT. The vibrating sensation in affections of the nervous system and in diabetes. *Lancet* 1905; **1**: 855–6.
8 Pavy FW. Introductory address to the discussion on the clinical aspect of glycosuria. *Lancet* 1885: 1085–7.
9 Pavy FW. On diabetic neuritis. *Lancet* 1904; **2**: 17–19, 71–3.
10 Buzzard T. Illustrations of some less known forms of peripheral neuritis; especially alcoholic monoplegia, and diabetic neuritis. *BMJ* 1890; **1**: 1419–22.
11 Rundles RW. Diabetic neuropathy: general review with report of 125 cases. *Medicine (Balt)* 1945; **24**: 111–60.
12 Thomas PK, Eliasson SG. Diabetic neuropathy. In: Dyck PJ, Thomas PK, Lambert EH, Bunge R (eds), *Peripheral Neuropathy*, 2nd edn. Philadelphia: W.B. Saunders, 1984: 1773–810.
13 Sindrup SH, Ejlertsen B, Gjessing H *et al*. Peripheral nerve function during hyperglycemic clamping in insulin-dependent diabetic patients. *Acta Neurol Scand* 1989; **79**: 412–18.
14 Gregersen G. Variations in motor conduction velocity produced by acute changes of the metabolic state in diabetic patients. *Diabetologia* 1968; **4**: 273–7.
15 Ward JD, Barnes CG, Fisher DJ, Jessop JD, Baker RWR. Improvement in nerve conduction following treatment in newly diagnosed diabetics. *Lancet* 1971; **1**: 428–30.

16 Valk GD, Nauta JJP, Strijers RLM, Bertelsmann FW. Clinical examination versus neurophysiological examination in the diagnosis of diabetic poly-neuropathy. *Diabetic Medicine* 1992; **9**: 716–21.

17 Feldman EL, Stevens MJ, Thomas PK, Brown MB, Canal N, Greene DA. A practical two-step quantitative clinical and electrophysiological assessment for the diagnosis and staging of diabetic neuropathy. *Diabetes Care* 1994; **17**: 1281–9.

18 Young MJ, Boulton AJM, Macleod AF, Williams DRR, Sönksen PH. A multi-centre study of the prevalence of diabetic peripheral neuropathy in the United Kingdom hospital clinic population. *Diabetologia* 1993; **36**: 150–4.

19 Walters DP, Gatling W, Mullee MA, Hill RD. The distribution and severity of diabetic foot disease: a community study with comparison to a non-diabetic group. *Diabetic Medicine* 1992; **9**: 354–8.

20 Barker RA, Macleod AF, Till AS, Lowy C, Sönksen PH. Awareness of foot problems in diabetic sensory neuropathy. *Practical Diabetes* 1992; **9**: 100–2.

21 Rydel A, Seiffer W. Untersuchungen über das Vibrationsgefühl oder die sog. 'Knochensensibilität' (Pallästhesie). *Arch Psychiatr Nervenkr* 1903; **37**: 488–536.

22 Liniger C, Albeanu A, Bloise D, Assal J Ph. The tuning fork revisited. *Diabetic Medicine* 1990; **7**: 859–64.

23 Semmes J, Weinstein S, Ghent L, Teuber HL. *Somatosensory Changes after Penetrating Brain Wounds in Man.* Cambridge, MA: Harvard University Press, 1960.

24 Holewski JJ, Stess RM, Graf PM and Grunfeld C. Aesthesiometry: quantification of cutaneous pressure sensation in diabetic peripheral neuropathy. *J Rehab Res Devel* 1988; **25**: 1–10.

25 Steiness I. Vibratory perception in diabetics. *Acta Med Scanda* 1963; **173** (Suppl 394): 1–91.

26 Lowenthal LM, Hockaday TDR. Vibration sensory thresholds depend on pressure of applied stimulus. *Diabetes Care* 1987; **10**: 100–2.

27 Guy RJC, Clark CA, Malcolm PN, Watkins PJ. Evaluation of thermal and vibration sensation in diabetic neuropathy. *Diabetologia* 1988; **28**: 131–7.

28 Bloom S, Till S, Sönksen PH, Smith S. Use of a biothesiometer to measure individual vibration thresholds and their variation in 519 non-diabetic subjects. *BMJ* 1984; **288**: 1793–5.

29 Macleod AF, Till AS, Lowy CL, Sönksen PH. Age corrected vibration threshold in diabetic subjects. *Diab Res Clin Pract* 1985; suppl 1: 351.

30 Boulton AJM, Hardisty CA, Betts RP, Franks CI, Worth RC, Ward JD, Duckworth T. Dynamic foot pressure and other studies as diagnostic and management aids in diabetic neuropathy. *Diabetes Care* 1983; **6**: 26–33.

31 Lindblom U. Quantitative testing of sensibility including pain. In: Stalberg E, Young R (eds), *Clinical Neurophysiology.* London: Butterworths, 1980: 169–90.

32 Masson EA, Veves A, Fernando D, Boulton AJM. Current perception thresholds: a new quick and reproducible method for the assessment of peripheral neuropathy in diabetes mellitus. *Diabetologia* 1989; **32**: 724–28.

33 Rendell MS, Dovgan DJ, Bergman TF, O'Donnell GP, Drobny EP, Katims JJ. Mapping diabetic sensory neuropathy by current perception threshold testing. *Diabetes Care* 1989; **12**: 636–40.

34 Fruhstorfer H, Lindblom U, Schmidt WG. Method for quantitative estimation of thermal thresholds in patients. *J Neurol Neurosurg Psych* 1976; **39**: 1071–5.

35 Dyck PJ, Zimmerman IR, O'Brien PC *et al.* Introduction of automated systems to evaluate touch-pressure, vibration and thermal cutaneous sensation in man. *Ann Neurol* 1978; **4**: 502–10.

36 Fowler CJ, Carroll MB, Burns D, Howe N, Robinson K. A portable system for measuring cutaneous thresholds for warming and cooling. *J Neurol Neurosurg Psych* 1987; **50**: 1211–15.

37 Armstrong FM, Bradbury JE, Ellis SH *et al.* A study of peripheral diabetic neuropathy. The implication of age-related reference values. *Diabetic Medicine* 1991; **8**: S94–S99.

38 Dorfman LJ, Bosley TM. Age-related changes in peripheral and central nerve conduction in man. *Neurology (Minneap)* 1979; **29**: 38–44.

39 Eccles JC. *The Physiology of Nerve Cells*. Baltimore, Md: The Johns Hopkins Press, 1969.

40 Panayiotopoulis CP, Scarpalezos S, Nastas PE. F-wave studies on the deep peroneal nerve. Part 1. Control Subjects. *J Neurol Sci* 1977; **31**: 319–29.

41 Lachman T, Shahani BT, Young RR. Late response as aids to diagnosis in peripheral neuropathy. *J Neurol Neurosurg Psychiat* 1980; **43**: 156–62.

42 Panayiotopoulis CP, Scarpalezos S. Chronodispersion of F-wave—a new method to detect abnormal motor nerve function. *Materia Medica Greca* 1976; **4**: 106–8.

43 Pirart J. Diabetes mellitus and its degenerative complications: a prospective study of 4,400 patients between 1947 and 1973. *Diabetes Care* 1978; **1**: 168–88, 252–63.

44 DCCT Research Group. The effect of intensive treatment of diabetes on the development and progression of long-term complications in insulin-dependent diabetes mellitus. *N Engl J Med* 1993; **329**: 977–86.

45 Dvornik D. *Aldose Reductase Inhibition*. New York: McGraw-Hill, 1987; 231.

46 Srivastava SK *et al.* Hyperglycaemia-induced activation of human erythrocyte aldose reductase and alterations in kinetic properties. *Biochem Biophys Acta* 1986; **870**: 302–11.

47 Gillon KRW *et al.* Sorbitol, inositol and nerve conduction in diabetes. *Life Sci* 1983; **32**: 1943–7.

48 Cameron NE *et al.* The effect of sorbinil on peripheral nerve conduction velocity, polyol concentrations and morphology in the streptozotocin diabetic rat. *Diabetologia* 1986; **29**: 168–74.

49 Schmidt RE, Plurad SB, Coleman B *et al.* Effects of sorbinil, dietary myo-inositol supplementation, and insulin on resolution of neuroaxonal dystrophy in mesenteric nerves of streptozoocin-induced diabetic rats. *Diabetes* 1991; **40**: 574–82.

50 Judzewitsch RG *et al.* Aldose reductase inhibition improves nerve conduction velocity in diabetic patients. *N Engl J Med* 1983; **308**: 119–25.

51 Boulton AJM, Levin S, Comstock J. A multicentre trial of the aldose-reductase inhibitor, tolrestat, in patients with symptomatic diabetic neuropathy. *Diabetologia* 1990; **33**: 431–7.

52 Macleod AF, Boulton AJM, Owens DR *et al.* A multicentre trial of the aldose-reductase inhibitor tolrestat, in patients with symptomatic diabetic peripheral neuropathy. *Diabetes & Metabolism* 1992; **18**: 14–20.

53 Low PA, Lagerlund TD, McManis PG. Nerve blood flow and oxygen delivery in normal, diabetic and ischemic neuropathy. *Int Rev Neurobiol* 1989; **31**: 355–438.

54 Newrick PG, Wilson AJ, Jakubowski J, Boulton ALM, Ward JD. Sural nerve oxygen tension in diabetes. *BMJ* 1986; **293**: 1053–4.

55 Tesfaye S, Malik R, Ward JD. Vascular factors in diabetic neuropathy. *Diabetologia* 1994; **37**: 847–54.

56 Stevens MJ, Feldman EL, Greene DA. The aetiology of diabetic neuropathy: the combined roles of metabolic and vascular defects. *Diabetic Medicine* 1995; **12**: 566–79.

57 Watkins PJ. Clinical observations and experiments in diabetic neuropathy. *Diabetologia* 1992; **35**: 2–11.

58 Foster AV, Eaton C, McConville DO, Edmonds ME. Application of Opsite film: a new and effective treatment of painful diabetic neuropathy. *Diabetic Medicine* 1994; **11**: 768–72.

59 Max MB, Lynch SA, Muir J *et al*. Effects of desipramine, amitriptyline, and fluoxetine on pain in diabetic neuropathy. *N Engl J Med* 1992; **326**: 1250–6.

60 Sindrup SH, Tuxen C, Gram LF, Grodum E, Skjold T, Brosen K, Beck-Neilsen H. Lack of effect of mianserin on the symptoms of diabetic neuropathy. *Eur J Clin Pharmacol* 1992; **43**: 251–5.

61 Sindrup SH, Gram LF, Brosen K, Eshoj O, Mogensen EF. The selective serotonin reuptake inhibitor paroxetine is effective in the treatment of diabetic neuropathy symptoms. *Pain* 1990; **42**: 135–44.

62 Stracke H, Meyer UE, Schumacher HE, Federlin K. Mexilitine in the treatment of diabetic neuropathy. *Diabetes Care* 1992; **15**: 1550–5.

63 Ewing DJ, Clarke BF. Diabetic autonomic neuropathy: present insights and future prospects. *Diabetes Care* 1986; **9**: 648–65.

64 Ewing DJ, Campbell IW, Clarke BF. The natural history of diabetic autonomic neuropathy. *Quart J Med* 1980; **193**: 95–108.

65 Sampson MJ, Wilson S, Karagiannis P, Edmonds M, Watkins PJ. Progression of diabetic autonomic neuropathy over a decade in insulin-dependent diabetes. *Quart J Med* 1990; **278**: 635–46.

66 Macleod AF, Smith SA, Cowell T, Richardson PR, Sönksen PH. Non-cardiac autonomic tests in diabetes: use of the galvanic skin response. *Diabetic Medicine* 1991; **8** (Symposium): S67–S70.

67 Giugliano MD, Marfella R, Quatraro A *et al*. Tolrestat for mild diabetic neuropathy. *Ann Intern Med* 1993; **118**: 7–11.

68 Neil HAW, Thompson AV, John S, McCarthy ST, Mann JI. Diabetic autonomic neuropathy: the prevalence of impaired heart rate variability in a geographically defined population. *Diabetic Medicine* 1988; **6**: 20–4.

69 Guy RJC, Richards F, Edmonds ME *et al*. Diabetic autonomic neuropathy and iritis: an association suggesting an immunological cause. *BMJ* 1984; **289**: 343–5.

70 Zanone MM, Petersen JS, Peakman M *et al*. High prevalence of autoantibodies to glutamic acid decarboxylase in longstanding IDDM is not a marker of symptomatic autonomic neuropathy. *Diabetes* 1994; **43**: 1146–51.

71 Barzilay J, Warram JH, Rand LI, Pfeifer MA, Krolewski AS. Risk for cardiovascular autonomic neuropathy is associated with the HLA-DR3/4 phenotype in Type I diabetes mellitus. *Ann Intern Med* 1992; **116**: 544–9.

72 McCulloch DK, Campbell IW, Wu FC, Prescott RJ, Clarke BF. The prevalence of diabetic impotence. *Diabetologia* 1980; **18**: 279–83.

73 Macleod AF, Smith SA, Sönksen PH, Lowy C. The problem of autonomic neuropathy in diabetic pregnancy. *Diabetic Medicine* 1990; **7**: 80–2.

74 Aagenaes Ö. *Neurovascular Examinations on the Lower Extremities of Young Diabetics, with Special Reference to Autonomic Neuropathy*. Copenhagen; C. Hamburgers Bogtrykkeri, 1962.

75 Watkins PJ. Facial sweating after food: a new sign of diabetic autonomic neuropathy. *BMJ* 1973; **1**: 583.

76 Horrocks PM, FitzGerald MG, Wright AD, Nattrass M. The time course and

diurnal variation of postural hypotension in diabetic autonomic neuropathy. *Diabetic Medicine* 1987; **4**: 307–10.

77 Ewing DJ, Martyn CN, Young RJ, Clarke BF. The value of cardiovascular autonomic function tests: 10 years experience in diabetes. *Diabetes Care* 1985; **8**: 491–8.

78 Smith SA. Reduced sinus arrhythmia in diabetic autonomic neuropathy: diagnostic value of an age-related normal range. *BMJ* 1982; **285**: 1599–1601.

79 Purewal TS, Watkins PJ. Postural hypotension in diabetic autonomic neuropathy: a review. *Diabetic Medicine* 1995; **12**: 192–200.

80 Wiles PG, Pearce SM, Rice PJS, Mitchell JMO. Vibration perception threshold: influence of age, height, sex and smoking, and calculation of accurate centile values. *Diabetic Medicine* 1991; **8**: 157–61.

81 Zhang WY, Li Wan Po A. The effectiveness of topically applied capsaicin. A meta-analysis. *Eur J Clin Pharmacol* 1994; **46**: 517–22.

82 Hansson S. Segmental median nerve conduction measurements discriminate carpal tunnel syndrome from diabetic polyneuropathy. *Muscle & Nerve* 1995; **18**: 445–53.

83 Barohn RJ, Sahenk Z, Warmolts JR, Mendell JR. The Bruns-Garland syndrome (diabetic amyotrophy). Revisited 100 years later. *Arch Neurol* 1991; **48**: 1130–5.

84 Moeser PJ, Kent JR. Diabetic amyotrophy without pain. A puzzling clinical picture. *Postgraduate Med.* 1991; **89**: 90–2.

7

Diabetic Foot

M. EDMONDS and A.V.M. FOSTER

Diabetic Department, King's College Hospital, London

INTRODUCTION

Foot ulceration is a leading cause of hospital admission for patients with diabetes and an extremely expensive complication of diabetes. The prevalence of foot ulceration in two community-based surveys in the United Kingdom was 5% in Oxford[1], and 7.4% in Poole[2], whereas the incidence of foot ulceration in a four-year follow-up study of 469 consecutive diabetic patients in Manchester UK, without previous history of foot ulceration, was 10.2%[3].

CLASSIFICATION AND DIAGNOSIS OF THE DIABETIC FOOT

INTRODUCTION

The feet are the target of peripheral neuropathy leading chiefly to sensory deficit and autonomic dysfunction. Ischaemia results from atherosclerosis of the leg vessels which in the diabetic is often bilateral, multisegmental and distal, involving arteries below the knee. Infection is rarely a sole factor but often complicates neuropathy and ischaemia. Nevertheless, it is responsible for considerable tissue necrosis in the diabetic foot.

For practical purposes, the diabetic foot can be divided into two entities: the neuropathic foot in which neuropathy predominates and there is a good circulation, and the neuroischaemic foot where there is both neuro-

Diabetic Complications. Edited by K. M. Shaw
© 1996 John Wiley & Sons Ltd

Table 7.1. Features of neuropathic and neuroischaemic feet

Neuropathic feet	*Neuroischaemic feet*
Features	*Features*
Warm	Cool
Foot pulses palpable (bounding)	Foot pulses impalpable
Veins on foot dorsum may be distended	Skin atrophic
Pink skin	Blanching on elevation; rubor on dependency
Complications	*Complications*
Callosities	Claudication
Painless ulceration	Ulceration (may be painful)
Digital gangrene	Digital gangrene
Charcot's joint	Rest pain
Neuropathic oedema	

pathy and absence of foot pulses. The purely ischaemic foot, with no concomitant neuropathy, is rarely seen in diabetic patients and its management is the same as for the neuroischaemic foot. The features and complications of both these types of feet are listed in Table 7.1.

Infection often complicates ulceration in both the neuropathic and neuroischaemic foot. The ulcers are portals of entry for bacteria and it is often a polymicrobial infection that spreads rapidly through the foot causing overwhelming tissue destruction[4]. Such tissue destruction is the main reason for major amputation in the neuropathic foot.

Recent studies have indicated that approximately 50% of the diabetic feet presenting to dedicated foot clinics are neuropathic and 50% neuro-ischaemic[4,5].

However, amputation is not an inevitable consequence of vascular disease or neuropathy. Early recognition of the 'at risk' foot, the prompt institution of preventive measures, and the provision of rapid and intensive treatment of foot complications in multidisciplinary foot clinics has reduced the number of amputations in diabetic patients[4,5].

In assessing the diabetic foot, it is important to consider the vascular and neurological status as well as mechanical pressures affecting the foot.

VASCULAR STATUS

The principal task in diagnosing the neuropathic or the neuroischaemic foot is to ascertain the presence or absence of pulses. The most important manoeuvre is thus the palpation of foot pulses, an examination which is often undervalued. If either of the pulses in the foot can be felt, i.e. posterior tibial or dorsalis pedis, then it is highly unlikely that there is significant ischaemia. Absence of both pulses in the foot indicates a reduction in circulation. This can be confirmed by measuring the pressure index which is the ratio of ankle systolic pressure to brachial systolic pressure. In normal subjects, the pressure index is usually >1, but in the presence of ischaemia is <1. Thus, absence of pulses and a pressure index of <1 confirms ischaemia. Conversely, the presence of pulses and a pressure index of >1 rules out ischaemia and this has important implications for management, namely that macrovascular disease is not an important factor and arteriography is not indicated.

However, between 5 and 10% of the total diabetic population have non-compressible peripheral vessels giving an artificially elevated systolic pressure, even in the presence of ischaemia. It is thus difficult to assess the diabetic foot when the pulses are not palpable, but the pressure index is >1. There are two explanations. The examiner may have 'missed' the pulses, particularly in an oedematous foot, and should go back to palpate the foot after the vessels have been located by Doppler ultrasound. If the pulses remain impalpable, then ischaemia probably exists in the presence of medial wall calcification. In these circumstances, blood velocity waveforms obtained by Doppler ultrasound should be examined and toe pressures measured.

The Doppler waveform becomes abnormal, distal to an obstructing lesion, with loss of normal rapid systolic upstroke and loss of diastolic flow. With diminishing flow, the waveform becomes flattened or 'damped' before it finally disappears. Several methods of signal analysis have been proposed to quantify changes in flow waveform and provide an index of severity of arterial disease[6].

Measurement of toe systolic pressure requires a toe cuff and a device for detecting toe blood flow, e.g. laser Doppler or a form of plethysmography. A toe pressure of 30 mmHg or less is indicative of severe ischaemia and a very poor prognosis[7].

Similarly, a transcutaneous oxygen pressure measured on the dorsum of the foot of less than 30 mmHg is also evidence of severe ischaemia[8].

NEUROLOGICAL STATUS

Neurological status can be assessed by detecting sensation to pinprick and cotton wool, and vibration using a 128 cps tuning fork starting at the distal foot and moving proximally to confirm a symmetrical stocking distribution of peripheral neuropathy. Knee and ankle jerks should be examined; their absence is evidence of peripheral neuropathy, although knee jerks are retained until surprisingly late. It is difficult to examine the autonomic nerves except to note a dry skin with marked fissuring as indicative of a sweating autonomic deficit.

Having diagnosed a neuropathy, it is important to ascertain whether the patient has lost protective pain sensation that would render him or her susceptible to foot ulceration.

Two clinical investigations are useful; vibrometry and nylon filaments. Vibration threshold can be measured using a hand-held Biothesiometer (Bio-medical Instrument Company, 15764 Munn Road, Newbury, Ohio 44065, USA). The vibration threshold increases with age, and values must always be compared with age adjusted nomograms.

Nylon monofilaments test the threshold to pressure sensation. These are of various diameters and can be obtained from Hanson's Disease Foundation Inc., Carville, LA[9]. The filament is applied to the foot until it buckles, when the patient is able to detect its presence. Buckling of the 5.07 monofilament occurs at 10 g of linear pressure and is the limit used to detect protective pain sensation. If the patient does not detect the filament, then protective pain sensation is assumed to be lost.

Thus the neuropathic foot is diagnosed in the presence of neuropathy and palpable pulses with a pressure index of >1, and the neuroischaemic foot in the presence of neuropathy and impalpable foot pulses.

Peripheral neuropathy in the foot leads to both somatic and autonomic damage. Small fibre neuropathy may initially dominate, with associated loss of pain and heat sensation. A 'pseudosyringomyelic' pattern may result in which loss of heat sensation is distal and length related[10], and pain and thermal sensation are lost before sensations of light touch or vibration[11].

Sympathetic denervation which is characteristic of diabetic neuropathy is also a result of small fibre loss[12]. A peripheral sympathetic defect has been documented by direct measurement of sympathetic activity in post-ganglionic C fibres in the diabetic neuropathic limb[13], and sympathetic nerve endings to small arterioles in the diabetic limb are either entirely absent or are found at a significantly greater distance from effector sites compared with controls[14].

Eventually a mixed fibre neuropathy develops in the diabetic foot involving both small and large sensory myelinated fibres with reduction in touch, vibration and proprioception sense as well as pain and temperature. Motor fibres are also affected with slowed motor conduction velocities and reduced or absent action potentials of the intrinsic muscles of the feet. This can lead to wasting and weakness of intrinsic foot muscles and subsequent deformity including claw toes, resulting in abnormal distribution of weight bearing as well as friction from footwear with subsequent ulceration (see below).

Diminished or absent sweating in the feet and legs commonly occurs in patients with diabetic neuropathy as a manifestation of peripheral sympathetic denervation. Indeed, anhidrosis of the feet may be responsible for cracking of the skin, resulting in a portal of entry for infections. The sweating loss normally occurs in a stocking distribution, which can extend into the trunk and above which there may be excessive sweating. Patchy sweating loss sometimes occurs.

PRESSURE

The presence of excessive pressure is a prerequisite for the development of a neuropathic ulcer. Cross-sectional studies have shown that foot pressures in neuropathic diabetic subjects are higher compared to non-neuropathic subjects and foot ulcers develop predominantly in areas of high pressure[15]. Recently, a prospective study has shown that high foot pressures are predictive of subsequent foot ulceration[16]. Plantar pressure can be measured with a number of commercially available systems. However, progress has not yet been reached to the point of positive identification of a threshold pressure at which ulceration would likely occur in an individual with loss of protective sensation. Furthermore, different systems for measuring pressure distribution yield different results in the same patient[17]. Elevated foot pressures are more likely to be present when the foot is deformed. The presence of neuropathy, even in its very earliest form with relatively mild sensory defects, may itself predispose to elevated foot pressures. Patients with foot ulcers tend to be heavier than others, although weight does not itself necessarily cause high foot pressure. Although vertical forces are obviously important, horizontal or shear forces must also be instrumental in damaging the neuropathic foot, and the sites of healed ulcers have been shown to correspond to the sites of maximal shear forces.

Shear forces are difficult to measure, and there are no commercially available instruments to measure shear force. However, recent interest has resulted in several groups attempting to measure this. The underlying principle is to use magneto-resistive elements attached to the sole and by this means horizontal shear forces can be measured. Tappin *et al*[18] were the first to describe the use of this technique for measuring discrete plantar stresses with a uniaxial shear transducer. Laing *et al*[19] have further developed Tappin's device by making it smaller in diameter and thickness. A triaxial transducer incorporating a biaxial shear stress section has been described by Lord *et al*[20] and this measures shear in two orthogonal directions. The transducer is mounted in an inlay which can directly replace the normal deep inlay of an extra depth shoe.

PREDISPOSING FACTORS TO ULCERATION IN THE
NEUROPATHIC AND NEUROISCHAEMIC FOOT

Having classified the foot into neuropathic and neuroischaemic entities, it is important to look for predisposing factors to ulceration, namely deformity, callus formation and oedema.

DEFORMITY

Deformities result in bony prominences which lead to areas of high localized pressure. The response to such pressure is different in the neuropathic foot compared with the neuroischaemic foot. In the neuropathic foot, the response to pressure is hyperkeratosis and callus formation with eventual ulceration. In the ischaemic foot, pressure leads to direct tissue damage and ulceration.

Charcot Deformity

Bony damage in the metatarsal–tarsal region leads to two classical deformities, the rocker bottom deformity, in which there is displacement and subluxation of the tarsus downwards, and the medial convexity, which results from displacement of the talonavicular joint or from tarsometatarsal dislocation. If these deformities are not accommodated in properly fitting footwear, ulceration at vulnerable pressure points often develops.

Hammer Toes

This is a flexion deformity of the proximal interphalangeal joint. It often leads to ulcer formation on the dorsal surface of the toes.

Claw Toes

These are characterized by hyperextension of the metatarsal phalangeal joints. They are often associated with pes cavus and callosities often develop over the dorsal surface of the toes and on the plantar surface of the metatarsal heads or the tips of the toes.

Although claw toes may be related to small muscle weakness secondary to neuropathy, they are often unrelated, especially when the clawing is unilateral and associated with trauma or surgery of the forefoot.

Pes Cavus

Normally the dorsum of the foot is domed due to the medical longitudinal arch which extends between the first metatarsal head and the calcaneus.

When it is abnormally high, the deformity is called pes cavus and the abnormal distribution of weight leads to excessive callus formation under the metatarsal heads.

Hallux Rigidus

This leads to stiffness of the first metatarsal phalangeal joint with loss of dorsiflexion and results in excessive forces on the plantar surface, causing callus formation.

Nail Deformities

Gross thickening or deformity of the nail is often seen in the neuropathic foot, and in severe cases of neuropathy, atrophy of the nail develops.

Ingrowing toe nails arise when the nail plate develops a convex deformity, putting pressure on the tissues at the nail edge. Callus builds up at the nail edge in response to the pressure and inflammation. As a result of ulceration and infection, usually after an episode of trauma, the nail penetrates into the flesh at the nail edge.

Deformities Related to Previous Trauma and Surgery

Deformities of the hip and fractures of the tibia or fibula lead to shortening of the leg and hence abnormal gait, which predisposes to foot ulceration.

Ray amputations are normally performed for digital sepsis in the neuropathic foot. They are usually very successful, but obviously disturb the biomechanics of the foot leading to high pressure under the metatarsal heads of the adjacent rays.

Deformities Related to Limited Joint Mobility

Limitation of joint motion secondary to glycation of connective tissues can lead to deformity and high plantar pressures. The normal foot has been described as a mobile adaptor and when mobility is impaired, elevated plantar pressure during walking results. Limitation of the ankle joint results in a fixed plantar flexion deformity (equinus) which leads to high mechanical loads under the forefoot[21].

CALLUS

Callus formation is common in the diabetic foot and also causes elevated plantar pressure. In a study of 17 patients peak plantar pressures were reduced after sharp debridement of callus by an average of 26%[22]. In addition, gait pattern is disturbed in patients with diabetic neuropathy and this may alter the foot pressure distribution, making the foot more prone to the effects of high pressures, again leading to callus formation[23].

OEDEMA

Oedema is a major factor predisposing to ulceration, in both the neuropathic and ischaemic foot, often exacerbating a tight fit inside poorly fitting shoes, which should also be examined.

The presence of foot oedema may not only underlie the development of foot ulcers when the shoes become too tight, but also could impede healing of established ulcers. Oedema is common in elderly patients, but in diabetic patients there are additional reasons for its occurrence, either from neuropathy or less commonly from fluid retention or nephrotic syndrome in patients with diabetic nephropathy.

Oedema is a complication of severe diabetic neuropathy. It has long been recognized and was observed in 35 of 125 patients with neuropathy described by Martin[24]. It is therefore not a rare phenomenon, although severe intractable oedema resulting from neuropathy is exceptional. This form of oedema probably results from the major haemodynamic abnormalities associated with neuropathy. Thus, the high blood flow, vasodilatation and arteriovenous shunting resulting from sympathetic denervation lead to abnormal venous pooling, and recently high venous pressures have been demonstrated in the neuropathic foot. Oedema probably develops because of loss of the venivasomotor reflex, which normally occurs on standing and results in an increase in precapillary resistance: the inability of the foot to compensate for the rise in venous pressure would thus predispose to oedema formation. Relief of oedema by administration of the sympathomimetic agent ephedrine[25] lends further strength to the argument that sympathetic failure is the cause of oedema.

COMPLICATIONS OF THE NEUROPATHIC FOOT

NEUROPATHIC ULCER

Presentation

The most frequent complication of the neuropathic foot is the neuropathic ulcer. Its classical position is under the metatarsal heads, but it is more frequently found on the tips of the toes (Figure 7.1) and occasionally on the dorsum of the toe, between the toes and on the heel. The neuropathic ulcer is usually surrounded by callus tissue and is generally painless. The

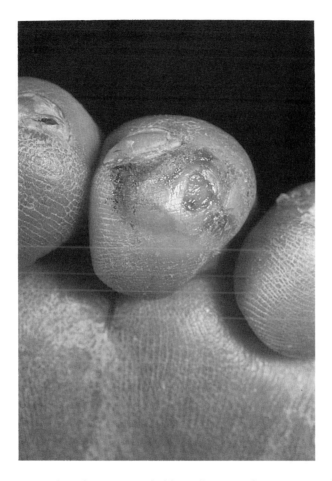

Figure 7.1. Neuropathic ulcer surrounded by callous on plantar aspect of third toe

ulcers on the plantar surface of the feet are usually circular, with a punched out appearance often penetrating to involve deep tissues including bone.

Neuropathic ulcers result from mechanical, thermal or chemical injuries that are unperceived by the patient because of loss of pain sensation. Loss of sensation, especially awareness of pain, is obviously a vital predisposing factor although autonomic neuropathy is also important. Motor neuropathy also plays a role with paralysis of the small muscles contributing to structural deformities such as claw toes. This leads to prominence of the metatarsal heads in the ulcerated foot.

Direct mechanical injuries may result from treading on nails and other sharp objects, but the most frequent cause of ulceration from mechanical factors is neglected callosity. This results from excess friction at the tips of the toes and from high vertical and shear forces under the plantar surface of the metatarsal heads on walking. The repetitive mechanical forces of gait eventually result in callosity formation, inflammatory autolysis and subkeratotic haematomas. The callosities are painless and are neglected by the patient. The presence of haemorrhage into a callus is a sign of early ulcer formation with a 50% chance of finding an ulcer when it is removed[26]. Tissue necrosis occurs below the plaque of callus resulting in a small cavity filled with serous fluid which eventually breaks through to the surface with ulcer formation.

At this stage, infection usually supervenes, caused by organisms from the surrounding skin which are usually *Staphylococcus aureus* or streptococci. If drainage is inadequate, cellulitis develops with spread of sepsis to infect underlying tendons, bones and joints. Occasionally staphylococci and streptococci are present together and these can combine to produce a rampant cellulitis that extends rapidly through the foot producing marked necrosis within only a few hours. Streptococci secrete hyaluronidase which facilitates widespread distribution of necrotizing toxins from staphylococci. Enzymes from these bacteria are also angiotoxic and cause *in situ* thrombosis of vessels. If both vessels are thrombosed in the toe, then it becomes necrotic and gangrenous, and this is probably the basis of so-called 'diabetic' gangrene in which tissue necrosis is seen only a few centimetres away from a bounding dorsalis pedis pulse. Aerobic Gram-negative organisms as well as anaerobic organisms flourish in deep-seated infections. Both aerobic and anaerobic organisms can rapidly infect the bloodstream and occasionally result in life-threatening bacteraemia.

Severe sepsis in the diabetic foot is often associated with gas in the soft tissues. Subcutaneous gas may be detected by direct palpation of the foot and the diagnosis is confirmed by the appearance of gas in the soft tissue on the radiograph. Although clostridial organisms have previously been held responsible for this presentation, non-clostridial organisms are more frequently the offending pathogens. These include *Bacteroides*, *Escherichia* and anaerobic streptococci.

Fungal infections also occur but usually do not cause systemic upset. However, infections of toe nails (tinea unguum) and interdigital spaces (tinea pedis) by such fungi as *Trichophyton* and *Candida albicans* can serve as portals of entry for bacteria.

In addition to mechanical injury, ulceration can also result from thermal or chemical injury. Thermal injuries cause direct trauma and damage to the epithelium. This often results from bathing feet in excessively hot water, from the injudicious use of hot water bottles, from resting the feet too close to a fire or radiator or from walking barefeet on hot sand during holidays in warm climates. Chemical trauma can result from the use of keratolytic agents such as 'corn plasters'. They often contain salicylic acid which causes ulceration in the diabetic foot.

Management of Neuropathic Ulceration

The management of ulceration in the purely neuropathic foot falls into three parts:

1. Removal of callus and local treatment

2. Eradication of infection

3. Reduction of weight-bearing forces.

Removal of callus
The callus which surrounds the ulcer must be removed by expert podiatry. Excess keratin should be 'pared' away with a scalpel blade to expose the floor of the ulcer and allow efficient drainage of the lesion and re-epithelialization from the edges of the ulcer. A simple non-adhesive dressing should be applied, after cleaning the ulcer and surrounding tissue with saline. Use of wound healing factors is being explored and recent studies have shown that it may speed healing in the neuropathic foot[27].

Eradication of infection
A bacterial swab should be taken from the floor of the ulcer after the callus has been removed. A superficial ulcer may be treated on an out-patient basis and oral antibiotics prescribed, according to the organism isolated, until the ulcer has healed. The patient should be instructed to carry out daily dressings of the ulcer.

If cellulitis or skin discoloration is present, the limb is threatened and urgent hospital admission should be arranged. The limb should be rested, and the ulcer irrigated with 2% Milton (sodium hypochlorite) solution. After blood cultures have been taken intravenous antibiotics are administered to treat possible staphylococci, streptococci, Gram-negative bacteria and anaerobes (flucloxacillin 500 mg 6 hourly, amoxycillin 500 mg IV 8 hourly, ceftazidime 1 g 8 hourly and metronidazole 1 g per rectum 8 hourly). This antibiotic regimen will need revision after the results of bacterial cultures are available. Blood glucose may need to be controlled with an intravenous insulin pump.

In the neuropathic foot, it is important that all necrotic tissue be removed and abscess cavities drained surgically. If gangrene has developed in a digit, a ray amputation to remove that toe and part of its associated metatarsal is necessary and is usually very successful in the neuropathic foot[4].

Reduction of weight bearing forces

Bedrest in the acute stages of ulceration is ideal and will obviously remove the weight bearing forces to promote healing. Proper care should be taken of the heels and foam wedges used to protect them from pressure in bed. However, bed rest is not always possible. In the short term, a total contact plaster cast (with minimum of padding) can be applied to 'unload' the ulcer and reduce shear forces[28]. Other forms of cast have become popular especially removable casts, such as the Scotch cast boot[29]. Padded hosiery may also help to relieve pressure. With regular rotation, these padded socks have been shown to reduce plantar pressures for at least 6 months[30]. In the long term, redistribution of weight bearing forces can be achieved by special footwear which is fashioned from casts of the patient's foot. Insoles made of closed cell polyethylene foams such as Plastazote have energy absorbing properties. These can be heated and moulded to the shape of the foot to cushion the plantar surface of the foot and to spread the forces of weight bearing evenly. When subject to wear and tear, Plastazote insoles can 'bottom out' and it is now possible to use more durable materials such as Poron. Indeed, composite insoles are often made with an upper layer of polyethylene foam for total contact and a lower layer of microcell rubber for resilience[31]. When there has been previous ulceration, a rigid weight distributing cradle is required, as well as cushioning, to relieve weight from high pressure areas and to transfer it to other less vulnerable areas. Traditionally, cork cradles have been used, but recently Plastazote cradles have been manufactured often with 'windows' cut out (and filled in with cushioning material such as Neoprene) for weight relief at these sites.

Moulded insoles must be accommodated in extra depth shoes. When the foot is not deformed, shoes fashioned from commercial lasts and available 'off the shelf' can be used. If the patient has a foot deformity with healed neuropathic ulcers, it is necessary to make individual lasts from casts of the patient's foot. In either case, the heels must be low, and slipping is prevented by using lace-ups. The forefoot should be broad and square and the uppers of high-quality leather which will adapt to toe pressure[32]. When pressure points are not adequately relieved by cushioned insoles, it is necessary to modify the soles of the shoe. When the ulcer is under the plantar surface of the first toe, a rigid rocker sole allows the shoe to rock like a see-saw on a pivot under the centre of the shoe minimizing contact between the forefoot and floor during gait. If the ulcer is under the metatarsal heads, a metatarsal bar placed just proximal to the heads can re-apportion weight bearing forces along the shafts.

CHARCOT FOOT

Presentation

The most frequent location of the neuropathic joint is the tarsal–metatarsal region, followed by the metatarsophalangeal joints and then the ankle and subtalar joints[33]. The initial presentation is often a hot, swollen foot which can be uncomfortable in up to one-third of cases and is often mis-diagnosed as cellulitis or gout. The precipitating event is usually a minor traumatic episode such as tripping. If the patient presents within a few days, radiographs are often normal, although isotope bone scans may be grossly abnormal with localized areas of high uptake representing excessive osteoblastic activity and heralding eventual radiological abnormalities. A common early radiological abnormality is fracture, which is followed by osteolysis, bony fragmentation and finally joint subluxation and disorganization. In addition to fracture, erosions, periosteal new bone formation and sclerosis are also prominent bony findings in the development of the Charcot joint. Sclerosis is usually associated with lucency in the heads of the metatarsals, the final appearance being similar to the Frieberg's infraction lesion associated with osteonecrosis of the epiphysis of the metatarsal head. These initial bony abnormalities eventually lead to secondary joint destruction with subluxation of the metatarsophalangeal joints, dislocation of the tarsal, subtalar and ankle joints, and fragmentation of bone and soft tissue calcification[34].

The process of destruction takes place over a few months only and leads to two classic deformities: the rocker bottom deformity, in which there is displacement and subluxation of the tarsus downwards, and the medial convexity, which results from displacement of the talonavicular joint or from tarsometatarsal dislocation. If these deformities are not accommodated in properly fitting footwear, ulceration at vulnerable pressure points often develops (Figure 7.2).

Pathogenesis

The development of Charcot osteoarthropathy depends on both peripheral autonomic and somatic defects. Recent studies have indicated a specific deficit of small fibre function[35]. Furthermore, an adequate blood supply is necessary and notably the development of the Charcot foot has been described in the foot after successful arterial bypass surgery[36]. It is suggested that the evolution is as follows. Sympathetic denervation of arterioles causes an increase of blood flow which in turn causes rarefaction of bone, making it prone to damage even after minor trauma. Bone formation and structure are closely linked with vascular changes. Large venules

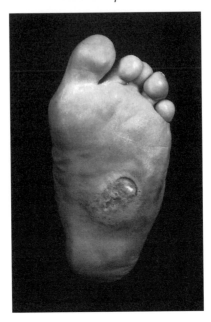

Figure 7.2. Ulceration of rocker bottom deformity under the Charcot foot

containing rapid linear velocities of blood flow cause resorption of bone spicules[37]. In animals, the site of maximum bone calcium loss after para-plegia corresponds to areas of maximum blood flow, which may lead to increased resorption of bone[38]. Histological studies of Charcot joints have shown marked increase in vascularity with vessel dilatation and trabecula resorption by large numbers of osteoclasts[39]. Thus, increased bony blood flow can lead to bony resorption and susceptibility to fracture. Loss of sensation from somatic neuropathy permits abnormal mechanical stresses to occur, normally prevented by pain. Relatively minor trauma can then cause major destructive changes in susceptible bone.

Management

It is essential to make the diagnosis early, before extreme joint destruction has taken place. The initial presentation of unilateral warmth and swelling in a neuropathic foot after an episode of minor trauma is suggestive of a developing Charcot joint.

There is no definite treatment that halts the progression of the disease, but immobilization may help. Treatment comprises rest (ideally bed rest), or the avoidance of weight bearing by the use of crutches until the oedema and local warmth have resolved. Alternatively, the foot can be put in a well-moulded non-walking plaster cast.

Immobilization is continued until bony repair is complete, usually a period of 2–3 months. Recently, bisphosphonates have been used to inhibit osteoclastic activity leading to a reduction in foot temperature and resolution of symptoms[40].

THE NEUROISCHAEMIC FOOT

PRESENTATION

The clinical features of ischaemia are intermittent claudication, rest pain, ulceration and gangrene. However, the most frequent symptom is ulceration. The ulcers present as areas of necrosis often surrounded by a rim of erythema. In contrast to ulceration in the neuropathic foot, callus tissue is usually absent. Furthermore, ulceration in the ischaemic foot is often painful although this varies from patient to patient according to the coexistence of a peripheral neuropathy. In the ischaemic foot, the most frequent sites of ulceration are the great toe, medial surface of the head of the first metatarsal (Figure 7.3), the lateral surface of the fifth metatarsal head and the heel.

PATHOGENESIS

The main factor responsible for a reduction in blood supply to the foot is atherosclerosis of the large vessels of the leg. In the diabetic subject, atherosclerosis is often multisegmental, bilateral and distal, involving tibial and peroneal vessels[41]. In the end stages, occlusion can be particularly extensive in the foot vessels[42]. Conversely, involvement of the aorto-iliac vessels is twice as common in non-diabetics as in diabetics.

Macrovascular Disease

Macrovascular disease in the diabetic leg can occur at the iliac, femoral, popliteal and tibial regions and this leads to a reduction in the perfusion of the foot. However, 40% of diabetic patients who have no pedal pulses and gangrenous lesions still have a palpable popliteal pulse, indicating patent iliac and femoral arteries[43].

In comparison with non-diabetics, diabetics have been noted to have a lower incidence of aorto-iliac disease, the same incidence of femoro-popliteal disease and a higher incidence of involvement of the arteries distal to

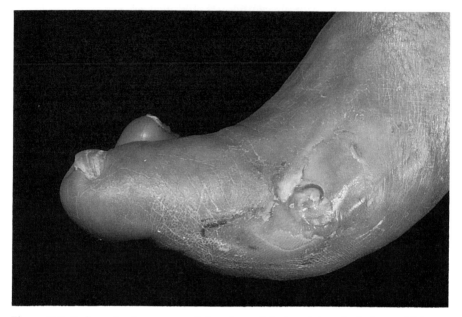

Figure 7.3. Ischaemic ulcer on medial surface of first metatarsal phalangeal joint

the popliteal artery[44]. The deep femoral artery is also more frequently diseased. The propensity for diabetics to have more diffuse vessel involvement tends to produce an unfavourable environment for the development of a satisfactory collateral circulation.

Two pathologies exist in the arteries of the diabetic leg and foot, atherosclerosis and medial wall calcification. The macroscopic features of streaks and plaques of atheroma are indistinguishable in diabetics and non-diabetics although the distribution is different[44]. They occur more frequently and at an earlier stage and appear to progress more rapidly in the diabetic patient. The actual pathology of the large vessel wall is not much different from that of the atherosclerotic non-diabetic artery. The intima is thickened by fatty deposits of cholesterol plaques which occur most commonly at bifurcations and the posterior wall of arteries and where the artery is constricted by muscle and fascia in the adductor canal. Whereas, the occlusive process frequently involves a single segment of an artery in the non-diabetic, atherosclerosis tends to be multisegmental in the diabetic.

Calcification of the tunica media of the muscular arteries is a common feature of longstanding diabetes. Medial calcification is much more common in diabetics, and its frequency has been related to age, male sex and duration of diabetes[45]. Neubauer made the interesting observation that calcification of the vessels of non-diabetics was related to higher levels of blood glucose following a glucose load[46]. Recent studies have linked calcification with neuropathy[47,48]. The effect of calcified vessels on the blood supply to the foot remains controversial. Arterial calcification is associated with a reduction in peak blood flow which is an index of the capacity of the circulation to increase[49]. However, other studies have shown no deficit in oxygen carrying power of the blood in patients with medial arterial calcification[50].

The distribution of macrovascular disease has been investigated both by morphological and arteriographic studies which indicate that the arterial disease of the lower extremities is different in diabetics and non-diabetics[51]. The main difference seems to be in the pattern of arterial occlusion, in that the distal arteries are apparently more severely affected in diabetes and are associated with calcification of the medial wall. The predilection to atherosclerosis for the vessels below the knee in diabetes is unexplained.

Microvascular Disease

So-called small vessel disease involving capillaries and arterioles had been thought to contribute substantially to impaired circulation in the feet. However, the significance of obliterative lesions of arterioles and capillaries with endothelial proliferation and basement membrane thickening is not known and the role, if any, in the development of ischaemic foot lesions remains to be elucidated. Although there is little evidence of an occlusive microvascular disease, functional abnormalities of the capillaries such as increased leaking of albumin from the capillaries to the interstitium may be important[52]. However, previous emphasis on small vessel disease in the diabetic foot has led to therapeutic nihilism and inappropriate care.

Ulceration and Gangrene

Tissue necrosis in the ischaemic limb is usually associated with minor trauma often complicated by infection. The traumas include direct pressure from tight shoes or socks, thermal and chemical injuries and injudicious cutting of the nails. When external pressures on localized areas of skin exceed capillary pressure, tissue necrosis follows. Initial incidents are often trivial and lead to trivial injuries. However, they are frequently neglected and rapidly lead to ulceration.

Minor trauma is often followed by infection. Ulcers serve as portals of entry for bacteria, and sepsis can rapidly spread through the foot. In the non-ischaemic foot, there is a good collateral circulation which can counteract major infection. In the diabetic ischaemic foot, obstructive disease is common in the metatarsal arteries[42] and this reduces communication in and between the plantar and dorsal arterial arches. The digital arteries are thus converted into 'end arteries'[53]. Many bacteria can elaborate angiotoxic substances which cause a septic thrombosis. Advancing infection can thus obliterate digital arteries and the tissue perfused by that artery becomes necrotic followed by rapid advancement of sepsis through the foot.

MANAGEMENT

Management can be divided into two parts: medical treatment and revascularization either by angioplasty or arterial reconstruction.

Medical

Medical management is indicated if the ulcer is small and shallow and is of recent onset within the previous month. Furthermore, it is the mainstay of treatment for those patients in whom reconstructive surgery is not feasible or possible because of widespread cardiovascular or cerebrovascular disease. Ischaemic ulcers may be painful and it may be necessary to prescribe opiates. It is the role of the podiatrist to remove necrotic tissue from the ulcers and, in the case of subungual ulcers, to cut back the nail to allow drainage of the ulcer. Ulcer swabs are taken as with the neuropathic foot and the ulcers are cleaned with normal saline and dressed with a sterile non-adherent dressing. It is important for the diabetologist to eradicate infection with prompt and specific antibiotic therapy after consultation with the microbiologist. However, severe sepsis in the ischaemic foot is an indication for emergency admission, first to control sepsis by intravenous antibiotics and surgical drainage, and secondly to assess the possibility of revascularization either by angioplasty or reconstruction. Footwear should be supplied to accommodate the foot and in most cases an extra depth ready-made shoe to protect the borders of the foot is adequate, unless there is severe deformity, when bespoke shoes will be needed. If any lesion, however small and apparently trivial, in the pulseless foot has not responded to conservative treatment within four weeks, then the patient should be considered for arteriography and revascularization; and in many cases, where there is severe ischaemia, referral will need to be initiated at a much earlier stage.

Revascularization

One of the most important advances in diabetic foot care has been the development of new techniques of revascularization of the ischaemic foot which has led to a reduction in the number of major amputations in diabetic patients. The economic cost of reconstruction is less than that of amputation[54] and successful revascularization has been associated with excellent mobility[55].

A modern vascular service is necessary to treat such arterial disease effectively, and this includes an imaging service to support complementary interventional radiology and surgical vascular management. The vascular service should carry out percutaneous catheter procedures, including angioplasty and thrombolysis, and bypass surgery including distal revascularization.

Modern vascular imaging includes conventional non-invasive Doppler ultrasound, to assess the pressure index and blood velocity pattern of the leg arteries, and Duplex ultrasound to give both anatomical and functional images. This is particularly useful in the assessment of the tibial and foot vessels. However, the gold standard is arteriography complemented by digital subtraction arteriography (DSA) which allows excellent views of the tibial and foot vessels.

Angioplasty

Recently, great advances have been made in percutaneous catheter techniques. Angioplasty balloons have been incorporated into guide wires and this has enabled lesions in the distal calf to be accessible to angioplasty[56]. Percutaneous catheter procedures including angioplasty have thus become established methods of treating peripheral vascular disease. Angioplasty is minimally invasive with a low mortality, low morbidity, needing short hospital stay and the techniques are repeatable. Given the same lesion, a diabetic patient will do equally well as a non-diabetic following femoral popliteal angioplasty, assuming equality of other factors, such as inflow or outflow[57]. There is a growing body of literature advocating angioplasty as the initial management of vascular disease where appropriate. The second report of the European Consensus on Critical Ischaemia recommends that, if angiography shows a technically suitable lesion and an experienced radiologist is available, a percutaneous catheter procedure should be tried as the first option even though surgery may eventually be needed. Furthermore, important adjunctive techniques to percutaneous balloon angioplasty have recently been developed, including thrombolytic therapy, which can be used to treat occlusions of up to one month's duration[58]. These can be used in diabetic patients, although the presence of proliferative retinopathy increases the risk of haemorrhage, and therefore a thorough ophthalmic assessment is necessary before this treatment.

Overall, it is important that early referral is made for catheter procedures before extensive tissue deficit has occurred. In these circumstances, experience has shown that a restoration of pulsatile blood flow is necessary from distal bypass surgery. Throughout such percutaneous procedures, it is extremely important to supervise the medical care of diabetic patients, who are often old and frail with impaired cardiac and cerebrovascular function. It is important that they do not get dehydrated, and if the serum creatinine is raised, renal function is protected by appropriate measures such as intravenous dopamine infusion (renal dose) during the procedures.

Arterial bypass

Recent advances in vascular surgery have led to the reappraisal of the optimum management of critical leg ischaemia, resulting in an expanded and successful role of arterial reconstruction in diabetic patients[59]. There has been an improved understanding of the pattern of atherosclerotic occlusion with an emphasis on arteriographic delineation of the distal arteries leading to success with distal arterial reconstruction. The microcirculation in the foot is not occluded in the diabetic patient[60], so that once the foot arteries are revascularized, excellent capillary perfusion results. Bypass grafting to infrapopliteal arteries for limb salvage is both technically feasible and durable with autogenous vein being superior to prosthetic grafts. In a group of unselected patients, including both diabetic and non-diabetic, patency rates were 72% in vein grafts and 51% in prosthetic grafts at follow-up after three years[55].

Recent reports have confirmed the value of the distal bypass in selected diabetic patients. Graft patency and limb salvage after 56 vein bypasses to the dorsal pedal artery resulted in actuarial graft patency and limb salvage of 92% and 98% respectively at 36 months[61]. Similar results have come from a further study in 72 diabetic patients with tibial artery disease reporting one- and five-year limb salvage rates of 81 and 72% respectively[62]. Thus, distal vein graft reconstruction for limb threatening ischaemia produces excellent patency rates and contributes significantly to limb salvage in these patients. The mean cost of primary arterial reconstruction is substantially cheaper than the cost of amputation. Distal bypasses are the most expensive of bypass surgery as further operations are sometimes needed during follow-up of the primary procedure, yet still their mean cost remains less than major amputation[55]. While under the care of the vascular service, the patient will need close medical supervision from the diabetologist and there should be close collaboration between the vascular surgeon, radiologist and diabetologist with a combined vascular X-ray conference providing an ideal forum for discussion and planning of treatment.

ORGANIZATION OF DIABETIC FOOT CARE: THE DIABETIC FOOT CLINIC

It is vital that there is close liaison between podiatrist, nurse, orthotist, physician and surgeon in the care of the diabetic foot; since 1981, diabetic foot problems have been treated with a special Diabetic Foot Clinic at King's College Hospital[4]. It has provided intensive chiropody, close surveillance, prompt treatment of foot infection and a footwear service by the attending shoe fitter. It has achieved a 50% reduction in major amputations by adhering to four main strategies:

1. To diagnose the specific lesions of the diabetic foot by means of a full clinical assessment, which can be divided into two parts: a medical history and examination, followed by a structured foot examination.

2. To treat the lesions of the foot rapidly and appropriately with a combined approach by podiatrist, diabetologist, and orthotist.

3. To provide regular and close follow-up of all lesions of the foot and within this follow-up to provide an emergency service to receive patients without appointment if they are concerned that their lesion has deteriorated or a new lesion has formed.

4. To prevent the redevelopment of foot problems in the patient who has recently healed. The aim is to prevent recurrence and, for the rest of the population to identify and educate those at high risk to prevent foot ulceration.

ROLE OF THE PODIATRIST

The podiatrist fulfils several important roles:

1. To carry out routine care of the neuropathic foot, including debridement of callus.

2. To perform debridement of the neuropathic ulcer. The callus that surrounds an ulcer needs regular removal by the podiatrist to promote re-epithelialization from the edge of the ulcer.

3. To apply the total contact cast. This is the most useful treatment for large indolent ulcers and is an effective way of keeping pressure off a plantar lesion while still enabling the patient to walk freely. This technique is effective as long as the cast is applied with great care and the patient returns early if problems arise.

4. To take care of the healed neuropathic ulcer. The site of a recently

healed neuropathic ulcer will continue to form callus very rapidly for several weeks and needs regular removal by the podiatrist.

5. To carry out aftercare of digital or ray amputation in the neuropathic foot. Large quantities of callus form around the edges of these wounds, and healing will be delayed if they are allowed to accumulate.

6. To carry out aftercare of skin grafts. Skin grafts on the plantar surface of the foot develop heavy hyperkeratosis that will break down if neglected. However, regular podiatry reduces callus and hyperkeratosis on grafts and will promote their survival.

7. To perform routine care of the neuroischaemic foot. Nails are cut straight across; thickened nails should be carefully and gently reduced with scalpel or nail drill. Any defects in the skin, no matter how small, should be carefully cleansed and dressed, avoiding the use of tape directly on the skin. The diabetic foot clinic is an ideal forum in which the podiatrists can work in dealing with the neuroischaemic foot, because constant assessment of the degree of ischaemia in conjunction with the diabetologist and vascular surgeon is always needed.

8. To treat ulceration in the neuroischaemic foot. Ischaemic ulcers are debrided by the podiatrist and sloughy tissue gently cut away without damage to viable tissue. They are not usually surrounded by callus but are associated with accumulations of slough that are gently cut away without damage being caused to viable tissue.

9. To facilitate autoamputation of necrotic toes. In the ischaemic foot it is often unwise to amputate toes, especially if the foot cannot be revascularized. Thus, a process of autoamputation is allowed. Debris and dried exudate and necrotic material are regularly pared away from the demarcation line by the podiatrist to facilitate this process.

10. To play an important part in the emergency service in conjunction with the diabetologist (see later discussion).

11. To educate the patients and their carers (see later discussion).

12. To advise on footwear. Podiatrists can advise patients that for everyday footwear, they should choose a shoe that fastens high on the foot with lace or strap, has an adequate toe box, and is sufficiently long, broad, and deep.

ROLE OF THE DIABETOLOGIST

1. To perform an initial assessment of patient with full medical history and examination, including a foot examination.

2. To diagnose the diabetic foot syndromes, particularly the neuropathic and neuroischaemic foot, and to examine the foot for deformities, oedema, lesions and signs of sepsis.

3. To diagnose the complications of the neuropathic foot and in cases of severe sepsis to arrange emergency admission and to start initial treatment with intravenous (IV) antibiotics and IV insulin, and to liaise with the surgeons regarding operative drainage and local amputation.

4. To assess the degree of ischaemia in the neuroischaemic foot and to diagnose its complications.

5. To form a plan of treatment for ulceration in the neuroischaemic limb. If it is not limb threatening, conservative treatment is employed. However, in cases of acute sepsis, it is necessary to arrange emergency admission, IV antibiotics, and IV insulin and to discuss management with the vascular surgeon. When there is worsening ischaemia, admission is arranged for urgent angiography.

6. To take part actively in the intensive follow-up service and to assess progress of all lesions, if necessary by assessing area from tracings on sterile film or by photography. If progress is not apparent, to re-examine the foot and plan appropriate adjustments to treatment.

7. To be responsible for all aspects of the management of sepsis in the diabetic foot, particularly early diagnosis, follow-up of the results of swabs, and the prescription of antibiotics.

8. To diagnose the causes of oedema in the diabetic foot and to prescribe appropriate treatment.

9. To achieve a wide experience in the manifestation and management of foot lesions. The presence of a surgeon in the actual diabetic foot clinic is rarely required on a regular basis, except to confirm the need for surgical intervention.

10. To take responsibility for all diabetic patients admitted from the foot clinic and, in conjunction with the surgeons, to ensure continuity of care while the patient is on the ward.

11. To take part in the education programme.

12. To be available to see and treat emergencies in conjunction with the podiatrist.

13. To make sure the patient is in good metabolic control.

ROLE OF ORTHOTIST

1. To redistribute weight bearing forces by special footwear. The orthotist supplies three main groups of shoes. Extra depth stock shoes are made in standard sizes but have an extra allowance in the depth dimension. They are fitted with sponge rubber insoles that can function as a cushion appliance or that can be replaced by purpose-made insoles of foot cradles. These shoes are available immediately from the orthotist and are suitable for patients with a history of ulceration but no great deformity. The second category is bespoke shoes for the deformed foot. The orthotist takes a plaster cast of the shape of the foot, and from this insoles or cradles, as well as the shoe itself, are fashioned. Often a rigid weight distributing cradle is needed to relieve weight from high pressure areas and to transfer it to other less vulnerable areas. The third category is temporary shoes made of felt or polythene foam. They are often supplied immediately to the patient while the bespoke shoes are constructed.

2. To follow up patients to check for patient acceptance of shoe and insole and to assess when new insoles and shoes are required.

3. To adjust shoes and insoles if new lesions develop.

4. To provide boots and special supporting braces to stabilize the ankle in the case of a Charcot joint.

Although the orthotist's formal visit is once weekly, it is possible to call him or her throughout the week particularly to supply temporary shoes when patients present as emergencies.

ROLE OF NURSE

Throughout the existence of the foot clinic, the nurse has had varying roles, partly depending on the interests of the individual nurse, although there has been a constant emphasis on education. In the early years, when there was one podiatrist only, the nurse assisted with foot dressings and education of the patients. When the number of podiatrists increased to two, the dressings were carried out by the podiatrists themselves after treatment of the foot ulcer. At present, the nurse manages the investigation room of the foot clinic, carries out neurological and vascular investigations, and also assists in the education of the patients.

Community nurses are welcome to visit the clinic and discuss their patients because this maintains an important line of communication with the community.

ROLE OF SURGEON

It is not necessary for the surgeon to attend the diabetic foot clinic regularly but to be available for consultation regarding difficult diagnoses or advanced foot problems that need to be treated in hospital. Thus, it is desirable for the surgeon to be in the out-patient area at the time of the foot clinic and to visit the clinic when necessary.

The main reasons for calling the surgeon are as follows:

1. To confirm the need for removal of infected bone in cases of chronic indolent ulceration with osteomyelitis.

2. To discuss cases of severe sepsis and soft tissue destruction that need surgical debridement and possible local amputation.

3. In the case of the ischaemic foot with severe limb threatening ischaemia, urgent referral should be made to the vascular surgeon to organize an inpatient treatment plan for treatment and investigation, including urgent angiography, in conjunction with the vascular radiologist.

The ultimate treatment is, of course, prevention, and this therapeutic approach must be through education of the patient in foot care and regular examination of the feet. It has been shown that patients who develop foot lesions have significantly less knowledge of diabetes, including foot care[63]. Moreover, it has been clearly shown that education reduces the number of major amputations in a diabetic clinic population[64]. Routine examination of the feet in diabetic patients is an important part of management in order to identify those at risk of ulceration, and to prevent its occurrence. However, it is a commonly underutilized preventive measure[65].

EMERGENCY COVER

An important part of the follow-up is to encourage patients to come to the clinic on an emergency basis if they are concerned that their lesion has deteriorated or a new lesion has formed. In a similar fashion, new patient referrals from podiatrists, physicians, and nurses are seen very quickly. The diabetic foot clinic at King's has an emergency service run by the podiatrist and the diabetologist where patients can be seen without an appointment as soon as they note a problem. In the first year, 107 patients were seen as emergencies: 83% of these had skin lesions, 14% had acute nail and joint lesions, and 3% had rest pain. Treatment of 86 of these patients was conducted entirely in the foot clinic and had a 90% healing rate; 21 patients with rampant sepsis were admitted without delay to achieve an 86% healing rate.

SCREENING

Screening technique is based on the foot examination described earlier, searching for the main risk factors, namely, neuropathy, ischaemia, deformity and oedema. High-risk patients then receive routine podiatry in the foot clinic, as well as education in foot care, in which regular examination of the feet by the patient and carers is stressed.

EDUCATION

The foot clinic has an important role not only in education of the patient but also in that of the health care professionals involved in foot care, including nurses, podiatrists, orthotists and physicians. All patients attending the clinic are instructed in basic foot care and further advice is given about danger signs and care of the patient's ulcer. The spoken word should be backed up by written advice.

CONCLUSION

Ulceration of the non-ischaemic diabetic foot depends on the presence of neuropathy, and is especially likely to occur in areas of the foot where high pressure (often associated with foot deformities) leads to the development of excessive callus which eventually breaks down and ulcerates.

Damage to small nerve fibres is the essential element of the neuropathy, causing loss of thermal and pain sensation, and sympathetic defects leading to diminished sweating and grossly altered haemodynamics. The arteries in the feet of these patients are rigid, and blood flow greatly increased both in skin and bones, causing both oedema and osteopenia; nutritive capillary flow remains unimpaired. Ulceration in the neuro-ischaemic foot results from pressure necrosis, often unperceived because of coexistent neuropathy. The main reduction in blood supply to the foot is related to atherosclerosis of the large vessels of the leg which, in the diabetic patient is often multisegmental, bilateral and distal, involving tibial and peroneal vessels.

The feet of diabetic patients must be carefully examined for the presence of deformities, callus formation, evidence of ischaemia and neuropathy in order to institute effective measures.

Optimal care of the diabetic foot is provided in a diabetic foot clinic where the skills of podiatrist, orthotist and nurse receive full support from physician and surgeon. Many lesions of the diabetic foot are avoidable and thus patient education is of immense importance.

REFERENCES

1 Neil HAW, Thompson AV, Thorogood M *et al.* Diabetes in the elderly: the Oxford community diabetes study. *Diabetic Medicine* 1989; **6**: 608–13.
2 Walters DP, Gatling W, Mullee *et al.* The distribution and severity of diabetic foot disease: a community study with a comparison to a non-diabetic group. *Diabetic Medicine* 1992; **9**: 354–8.
3 Young MJ, Bready JL, Veves A *et al.* The prediction of diabetic neuropathic foot ulceration using vibration perception thresholds: a prospective study. *Diabetes Care* 1994 (in press).
4 Edmonds ME, Blundell MP, Morris HE *et al.* Improved survival of the diabetic foot: impact of a foot clinic. *Quart J Med* 1986; **232**: 763–71.
5 Thomson FJ, Veves A, Ashe H *et al.* A team approach to diabetic foot care—the Manchester experience. *The Foot* 1991; **1**: 75–82.
6 Sidaway AN, Curry KM. Non invasive evaluation of the lower extremity arterial system. In: Frykberg RG (ed.), *The High Risk Foot in Diabetes Mellitus*. Edinburgh: Churchill Livingstone, 1991; 241–54.
7 European Working Group on Critical Leg Ischaemia. Second European Consensus Document on Chronic Critical Leg Ischaemia. *Eur J Vasc Surg* 1992; **6** (suppl A).
8 Jacobs MJHM, Ubbink D. Th, Kitslaar PJEHM *et al.* Assessment of the microcirculation provides additional information in critical limb ischaemia. *Eur J Vasc Surg* 1992; **6**: 135–41.
9 Birke JA, Sims DS. Plantar sensory threshold in the ulcerative foot. *Lepr Rev* 1986; **57**: 261–7.
10 Said B, Slama G, Selva J. Progressive centripetal degeneration of axons in small fibre type diabetic polyneuropathy. A clinical and pathological study. *Brain* 1983; **106**: 791–807.
11 Guy RJG, Clark CA, Malcolm PN, Watkins PJ. Evaluation of thermal and vibration sensation in diabetic neuropathy. *Diabetologia* 1985; **28**: 131–7.
12 Watkins PJ and Edmonds ME. Sympathetic nerve failure in diabetes. *Diabetologia* 1983; **25**: 73–7.
13 Fagius J. Microneurographic findings in diabetic polyneuropathy with special reference to sympathetic nerve activity. *Diabetologia* 1982; **23**: 415–520.
14 Imparato AM, Kim GE, Thomas PK. Abnormal innervation of the lower limb epineurial arterioles in human diabetes. *Diabetologia* 1981; **20**: 31–8.
15 Cavanagh PR, Ulbrecht JS. Clinical plantar pressure measurement in diabetes: rationale and methodology. *The Foot* 1994 (in press).
16 Veves A, Murray HJ, Young MJ, Boulton AJM. The risk of foot ulceration in diabetic patients with high foot pressure: a prospective study. *Diabetologia* 1992; **35**: 660–63.
17 Cavanagh PR, Ulbrecht JS. Plantar pressure in the diabetic foot. In: Sammarco GJ (ed.), *The Foot in Diabetes*. Philadelphia: Lea and Febiger, 1991; 54–70.
18 Tappin JW, Pollard J, Bechett EA. Method of measuring shear forces on the sole of the foot. *Clin Phys Physiol Meas* 1980; (1): 83–5.

19 Laing P, Deogan H, Cogley D *et al.* The development of the low profile Liverpool shear transducer. *Clin Phys Physiol Meas* 1992; **13**: 115–24.

20 Lord M, Hosein R, Williams RB. Method for in shoe shear stress management. *J Biomed Eng* 1992; **14**: 181–6.

21 Cavanagh PR, Ulbrecht JS. Biomechanical aspects of foot problems in diabetes: In: Boulton AJM, Connor H and Cavanagh PR (eds), *The Foot in Diabetes*. Chichester: John Wiley, 1994; 25–35.

22 Young MJ, Cavanagh PR, Thomas G, Johnton MM, Murray H, Boulton AJM. The effect of callus removal on dynamic plantar foot pressures in diabetic patients. *Diabetic Medicine* 1992; **9**: 55–7.

23 Cavanagh PR, Derr JA, Ulbrecht JS, Maser RE, Orchard TJ. Problems with gait and posture in neuropathic patients with insulin dependent diabetes mellitus. *Diabetic Medicine* 1992; **9**: 469–74.

24 Martin MM. Diabetic neuropathy. *Brain* 1953; **76**: 594–624.

25 Edmonds ME, Archer AG, Watkins PJ. Ephedrine: a new treatment for diabetic neuropathic oedema. *Lancet* 1983; **1**: 54–5.

26 Rosen RC, Davids MS, Bohanske LM. Haemorrhage into plantar callus and diabetes mellitus. *Cutis* 1985; **35**: 339–41.

27 Krupski WC, Reilly LM, Perez S, Moss KM, Crombleholme PA, Rapp JH. A prospective randomized trial of autologous platelet derived wound healing factors for the treatment of chronic non healing wounds: a preliminary report. *J Vasc Surg* 1991; **14**: 526–36.

28 Mueller MJ, Diamond JE, Sinacore DR *et al.* Total contact casting in treatment of diabetic plantar ulcers. *Diabetes Care* 1989; **12**: 384–8.

29 Burden AC, Jones GR, Jones R, Blandford RL. Use of the 'Scotchcast boot' in treating diabetic foot ulcers. *BMJ* 1983; **286**: 1555–7.

30 Veves A, Masson EA, Fernando DJS, Boulton AJM. Studies of experimental hosiery in diabetic neuropathic patients with high foot pressures. *Diabetic Medicine* 1990; **7**: 324–6.

31 Chantelau E and Leisch A. Footwear, uses and abuses. In: Boulton AJM, Connor H and Cavanagh PR (eds), *The Foot in Diabetes*. Chichester: John Wiley, 1994; 99–108.

32 Tovey FI. Establishing a diabetic shoe service. *Practical Diabetes* 1985; **2**: 5–8.

33 Sanders LJ, Frykberg RG. Diabetic neuropathic osteoarthropathy: the Charcot foot. In: Frykberg RG (ed.), *The High Risk Foot in Diabetes*. New York: Churchill Livingstone, 1991; 227–38.

34 Sinha S, Munichoodappa CS, Kozak GP. Neuroarthropathy (Charcot joints) in diabetes mellitus. *Medicine (Baltimore)* 1972; **51**: 191–210.

35 Stevens MJ, Edmonds ME, Foster AVM, Watkins PJ. Selective neuropathy and preserved vascular responses in the diabetic Charcot foot. *Diabetologia* 1992; **35**: 148–54.

36 Edelman SV, Kosofsky EM, Paul RA, Kozak GP. Neuro-osteoarthropathy (Charcot's Joint) in diabetes mellitus following revascularisation surgery: three case reports and a review of the literature. *Arch Intern Med* 1987; **147**: 1504–8.

37 McClugage SG, McCuskey RS. Relationship of the microvascular system to bone resorption and growth in situ. *Microvasc Res* 1973; **6**: 132–4.

38 Verhas M, Martinello Y, Mone M *et al.* Demineralisation and pathological physiology of the skeleton in paraplegic rats. *Calcif Tissue Int* 1980; **30**: 83–90.

39 Brewer AC, Allman RM. Pathogenesis of the neurotrophic joint: neurotraumatic vs neurovascular. *Radiology* 1981; **139**: 349–54.

40 Selby PL, Young MJ, Boulton AJM. Bisphosphonates—a new treatment for diabetic Charcot arthropathy. *Diabetic Medicine* 1994; **11**: 28–31.

41 Strandness DE Jr, Priest RE, Gibbons GE. Combined clinical and pathologic study of diabetic and non diabetic peripheral arterial disease. *Diabetes* 1964; **13**: 366–72.

42 Ferrier RM. Radiologically demonstrable arterial calcification in diabetes mellitus. *Aust Ann Med* 1967; **13**: 222–6.

43 Tooke JE. The impact of diabetes mellitus on extremity ischaemia. In: Kempczinski, RF (ed.), *Ischaemic Leg*. Year Book Medical Publishing. Chicago 1985; 51–69.

44 Warren S, Le Compte PM, Legg MA. *The pathology of Diabetes Mellitus*. Philadelphia: Lea and Febiger, 1966.

45 Ferrier TM. Radiologically demonstrable arterial calcification in diabetes mellitus. *Aust Ann Med* 1964; **13**: 222–8.

46 Neubauer B. A quantitative study of peripheral arterial calcification and glucose tolerance in elderly diabetics and non diabetics. *Diabetologia* 1971; **7**: 409–13.

47 Edmonds ME, Morrison N, Laws, Watkins PJ. Medial arterial calcification and diabetic neuropathy. *BMJ* 1982; **284**: 928–30.

48 Young MJ, Adams JE, Anderson GF, Boulton AJM, Cavanagh PR. Medial arterial calcification in the feet of diabetic patients and matched non diabetic control subjects. *Diabetologia* 1993; **36**: 615–21.

49 Christensen NJ. Muscle blood flow, measured by xenon and vascular calcifications in diabetics. *Acta Med Scand* 1968; **183**: 449–54.

50 Chantelau E, Ma XY, Herrnberger S, Dohmen C, Trappe P, Baba T. Effect of medial arterial calcification on O_2 supply to exercising diabetic feet. *Diabetes* 1990; **39**: 513–16.

51 Wheelock FC, Gibbons GW, Marble A. Surgery in diabetes. In: Marble A, Krall LP, Bradley RF, Christlieb AR, Soeldner JS (eds), *Joslin's Diabetes Mellitus*. Philadelphia: Lea and Febiger, 1985; 712–31.

52 Parving HH and Rasmussen SM. Transcapillary escape rate of albumin and plasma volume in short and long term juvenile diabetes. *Scand J Clin Lab Invest* 1973; **32**: 81–7.

53 O'Neal LW. Surgical pathology of the foot and clinicopathologic correlations. In: Levin ME and O'Neal LW, Bowker JH (eds), *The Diabetic Foot*. St Louis: CV Mosby, 1993; 457–91.

54 Cheshire NJW, Wolfe JHN, Noone MA. The economics of femorocrural reconstruction for critical leg ischaemia with and without autologous vein. *J Vasc Surg* 1992; **15**: 167–75.

55 Cheshire NJW, Wolfe JHN. Critical leg ischaemia: amputation and reconstruction. *BMJ* 1992; **304**: 312–15.

56 Bakal C, Sprayregen S, Scheinbaum K *et al*. Percutaneous transluminal angioplasty of the infra popliteal arteries, results in 53 patients. *Am J Radiol* 1990; **154**: 171–4.

57 Davies AH, Cole SE, Magee T *et al*. The effect of diabetes mellitus on the outcome of angioplasty for lower limb ischaemia. *Diabetic Medicine* 1992; **9**: 480–1.

58 Traughber PD, Cook PS, Micklos TJ *et al*. Intra-arterial fibrinolytic therapy for popliteal and tibial artery obstruction. *Am J Radiol* 1987; **149**: 453–6.

59 Logerfo FW, Gibbons GW, Pomposilli B Jr. Trends in the care of the diabetic foot. *Arch Surg* 1992; **127**: 617–21.

60 Logerfo FW, Coffman JD. Vascular and microvascular disease of the foot in diabetes. *N Engl J Med* 1984; **311**: 1615–19.
61 Tannenbaum G, Pomposelli GB, Maraccio EJ. Safety of vein bypass grafting to the dorsal pedal artery in diabetic patients with foot infection. *J Vasc Surg* 1992; **15**: 982–90.
62 Woelfle KD *et al*. Distal vein graft reconstruction for isolated tibio-peroneal occlusive disease in diabetics with critical foot ischaemia. How does it work? *Eur J Vasc Surg* 1993; **7**: 409–13.
63 Delbridge L, Appleberg M, Reeve TS. Factors associated with the development of foot lesions in the diabetic. *Surgery* 1983; **93**: 78–82.
64 Assal J-P, Gfeller R, Ekoe J-M. Patient education in diabetes. In: Bostrum H, Ljungstedt N (eds), *Recent Trends in Diabetes Research*. Stockholm: Almqvust & Wiksell 1981; 276–90.
65 Bailey TS, Yu HM, Rayfield EJ. Patterns of foot examination in a diabetes clinic. *Am J Med* 1985; **78**: 371–4.

8

Macrovascular Disease in Diabetes

K.M. SHAW

Department of Diabetes and Endocrinology,
Queen Alexandra Hospital, Portsmouth

INTRODUCTION

Diabetes exerts its greatest impact throughout the vascular system. This effect includes the well-described consequence of small vessel disease leading to serious complications including retinopathy, nephropathy and neuropathy, but also a substantial predisposition to premature and accelerated disorder of large blood vessels, macrovascular disease. Indeed the consequences of large disease now contribute not only to significant reduction in the quality of life of the person with diabetes, but also to the most likely cause of death. This is particularly so as advances in the management of microvascular disease now offer the real prospect that mortality and morbidity from these more specific complications of diabetes can be substantially lessened. For instance, a major cause of premature mortality in insulin-dependent diabetes over the years has resulted from nephropathy and end stage renal failure, but there is now clear evidence that the relentless progression to renal failure in such cases can be contained and indeed prevented. While advanced complications from microangiopathy are potentially preventable, the ravages of large vessel disease[1], particularly affecting the coronary, cerebral and peripheral circulation, continue unabated, now contributing to a much greater and disproportionate effect on overall health and longevity in people with diabetes.

Susceptibility to large vessel disease is increased substantially with both insulin-dependent diabetes (IDDM) and non-insulin-dependent diabetes (NIDDM). The development of large vessel disease is accelerated with IDDM, and often present at diagnosis with NIDDM. It is uncertain whether there are actual differences between the type of large vessel disturbance between IDDM and NIDDM. Apparent differences probably relate to different patterns of presentation for in the past microangiopathy has often been predominant with IDDM, while the manifestations of large vessel disease are more apparent in the NIDDM. As the impact of microangiopathy in IDDM lessens, it is quite likely that large vessel problems in IDDM will be seen to have the same degree of serious consequence as with NIDDM.

The effects of diabetes on the large vessels are seen predominantly at three major sites of the cardiovascular system, namely the coronary, cerebral and peripheral arteries. Such is the process that all three sites of the circulation are usually uniformly affected, conferring a triple susceptibility to arterial disease. Although the first clinical manifestation of such is often a specific event such as myocardial infarction, transient ischaemic episode or foot ulcer, almost certainly the initial clinical manifestation reveals the overall presence of generalized and diffuse arterial problems. Quite frequently symptoms of ischaemia from differing parts of the circulation are present together, and indeed pose management considerations when treatments are being planned. For instance, the person with claudication of the legs as a consequence of peripheral arterial disease often gives a simultaneous history of exertional angina, only limited by the restricted mobility. If revascularization is to be considered, the problem is posed as to which should be tackled first, for relief of one then carries the prospect of aggravation of the other. It can, therefore, be understood that management of one particular type of large vessel disorder has to take into account the effect on other aspects which can make treatment strategies very complicated. Furthermore, even medical therapies that may be of benefit for one disorder may disadvantage another. A classical example would be the use of beta blockers for angina and hypertension, which can seriously aggravate cold peripheries and claudication of the legs.

Undoubtedly, large vessel disease in diabetes is likely to become an increasing management problem, not only with NIDDM where the consequences have been only too evident, but also with IDDM as the consequences of microangiopathy become more effectively controlled. Although large vessel disease is not specific to diabetes, it is greatly increased in the presence of such. However, a widespread occurrence of arterial disease within the non-diabetic population does permit parallel observations to be made on the nature of the disturbance and the mechanisms contributing to its development. It is interesting that the most serious expression of large vessel disease with diabetes occurs most commonly where there is a high background instance of such in the population, which allows consideration of epidemiological factors to be made. Differences in population risk would seem to be predominantly geographical, providing potential clues as to why risk varies. For instance, the prevalence of coronary heart disease in Japan is known to be relatively small, and that reduced risk is shared by those with diabetes living in Japan. However, second generation Japanese with diabetes living in the USA develop severe coronary heart disease, presumed due to significant change in lifestyle or environment. Susceptibility to large vessel disease is determined by a complex interaction of various factors including hereditary predisposition, disturbance of metabolic state, and exposure to risk factors within the environment.

NATURE OF MACROVASCULAR DISEASE

The predominant large vessel disturbance of diabetes is that of atherosclerosis[2]. Considerable debate has been made concerning whether there are specific features to diabetes, or whether it is simply an exaggeration of that seen with the non-diabetic population. Overall there is probably no major qualitative difference in the type of atherosclerosis between diabetes and non-diabetes; it is predominantly an increase in the amount, extent and distribution. With diabetes, atherosclerosis is observed to be more extensive throughout the circulation with more distal involvement of blood vessels. In general, no specific arterial lesion with diabetes is seen, but there is evidence of more fatty streaks, intimal plaques and calcification of vessels. The process of atherosclerosis is probably similar to that observed in non-diabetes, with smooth muscle cell proliferation, intimal thickening, excess collagen production and medial calcification leading to reduced blood flow.

Having recognized that the essential atherosclerotic process probably follows a similar pattern to that with non-diabetes, some explanation for the increased susceptibility with diabetes must be evident. The possibility of a separate diabetic macroangiopathy, independent of but occurring in association with accelerated atherosclerosis, has been suggested, but it seems likely that some aspect of the disturbed metabolism in diabetes triggers and sustains the sequence leading to atherosclerotic change. Certain growth factors that can stimulate smooth muscle cell proliferation within blood vessels have been identified in serum from diabetic patients. Changes in platelet activity with increased adhesiveness and tendency to aggregation have also been observed, although it is not always easy to distinguish between primary alterations as a consequence of diabetes, from those changes known to occur secondarily in the presence of occlusive arterial disease. It is possible that diabetes leads to some alteration or disturbance of the endothelial barrier thus exposing sub-intimal tissue to platelet adhesion, which in turn stimulates smooth muscle cell activity and increased uptake of low density lipoprotein cholesterol.

EPIDEMIOLOGY

Variations in susceptibility to large vessel disease with diabetes may have a genetic basis, result from differing metabolic disturbance of the diabetes, of which the level of glycaemic control has long been a fundamental consideration, and many other associated risk factors, be they indicators of risk or truly causal. Some of these risk factors may in turn be directly dependent on disturbance of the diabetic state such as hyperlipidaemia, glycosylation and alterations of blood constituents including platelet adhesiveness. Other factors may be part of a clinical predisposition such as hypertension and obesity, while others may be truly avoidable factors such as cigarette smoking, poor diet or sedentary activity. The differing geographical susceptibility has already been mentioned in the case of the Japanese and, in general, expression of large vessel problems, particularly coronary heart disease, does correlate with the degree of atherosclerotic disease within the population concerned. However, varying prevalence between different communities living within the same regional area can also be identified, although differing genetic susceptibility cannot necessarily be presumed for there may be real differences in lifestyle such as diet or indeed physical activity. The increased risk of second generation Japanese in the USA would seem to be predominantly of a dietary nature.

Epidemiological studies do not always clearly distinguish IDDM from NIDDM and so it is not entirely certain to what extent there are real differences in predisposition between these two main types of diabetes. To some extent insulin-dependent diabetes is a more well-defined type of diabetes, characterized by genetic predisposition and autoimmune disturbance, while NIDDM appears to be a more heterogeneous disorder including, to variable extent, the more complex syndrome characterized by the constellation of central obesity, hypertension, impaired glucose tolerance and hyperlipidaemia. Because of the association of this syndrome with serious risk of large vessel disease, these features have sometimes been known as 'the deadly quartet'.

Some distinction between IDDM and NIDDM seems evident from the degree of disturbed glycaemic control that correlates with the development of arterial problems. Microangiopathy seems primarily related to the degree of hyperglycaemia and its duration, with an uncertain genetic factor. This may well be similar in both IDDM and NIDDM. For macro-angiopathy the situation is less clear. By its very nature IDDM predominantly presents at a younger age than NIDDM and so the opportunity for pre-clinical development of vascular disturbance is less. It is unusual to see serious arterial problems with teenage diabetes, or with a few years' duration. However, serious problems, including premature coronary disease, may present even as young as the mid-twenties, and is certainly detected increasingly during the third and fourth decades. With IDDM a distinct threshold of hyperglycaemia predisposing to microangiopathy around 11 mmol/l, is apparent, while the threshold for large vessel disease is clearly lower, possibly around 7 mmol/l, probably with increasing linear risk the higher the mean blood sugar levels. It is, however, unclear, to what extent hyperglycaemia[3] is a primary factor contributing to susceptibility or alternatively, simply a marker of other disturbed factors.

With NIDDM large vessel susceptibility is undoubted and substantial. So often the disease process is evident at the time the diabetes is diagnosed. An ischaemic toe may provide the first awareness of underlying diabetes, or an acute event such as myocardial infarction may unmask an underlying diabetic disposition. It is well known that the development of NIDDM is insidious and the process has often been developing subclinically for many years prior to diagnosis. During these years, while 'the clock is ticking' vascular disease may become established, accelerated and advanced. The fact that the actual disturbance of blood sugar levels itself may not be that severe during these years argues against a direct consequence of poor diabetic control, and with the NIDDM at least there is no clear correlation between severity and duration of hyperglycaemia. Often the glycaemic disturbance seems relatively slight, and yet even sugars in the category of impaired glucose tolerance may be associated with severe large vessel disease. As already mentioned, NIDDM may cluster with other known cardiovascular risk factors, suggesting a possible common aetiology, and forming an apparent syndrome (Syndrome X or Reavens Syndrome)[4] including other risk factors[5] such as hypertension and hyperlipidaemia, which will have their own aggravating effect on cardiovascular risk.

Epidemiological studies of considerable interest have arisen from observation that nutrition during the early stages of life, particularly *in utero* and during the first year of infancy, may predispose to ill-health in adulthood. In particular low birth weight[6] and reduced infant growth during the first year of life correlate with future development of impaired glucose tolerance, non-insulin-dependent diabetes, hypertension and susceptibility to coronary heart disease. It has been postulated that undernutrition in early life predisposes, indeed programmes, to increased prevalence of both maturity onset diabetes and coronary heart disease in adults. The precise means whereby such observations may be explained are uncertain, but it does seem as though birth weight and growth during early infancy are strong indicators of future risk of developing diabetes and coronary heart disease. However, such could only contribute in part to causation, and would not explain acquired risk, as say seen with geographical migration.

MECHANISMS AND RISK FACTORS

The cause of increased atherosclerotic risk in diabetes is multifactorial. From understanding the processes involved in the development of atherosclerosis, along with epidemiological observations, a number of factors associated with susceptibility to premature arterial disease have been identified. Debate occurs as to whether these factors are simply coincidental correlations or whether they truly contribute to the pathogenesis of arterial disease. As already discussed, no greater uncertainty exists than that observed with glycaemic control[3]. With IDDM some evidence exists that the degree of cardiovascular disorder is proportional to the preceding severity of hyperglycaemia, but certainly with NIDDM severe arterial disease may be associated with relatively moderate degrees of glucose intolerance. Good glycaemic control does not guarantee protection from development of large vessel disorder and once such circulatory problems are evident often at diagnosis with the NIDDM, there is no definite evidence that tightening of diabetic control alters outcome. The Diabetes Control and Complications Trial Research Group (DCCT)[7] reported on the effect of intensive treatment of diabetes on the development and progression of long-term complications in insulin-dependent-diabetes. The total of 14 041 patients with IDDM divided into two groups, a primary prevention cohort without pre-existing complications and a secondary prevention cohort of those with early complications, were studied over a mean period of 6.5 years. Each group was randomly assigned to either a conventional treated group or to a much more intensive therapeutic regimen. The effect on microvascular complications was striking, with substantial reduction in the development of retinopathy, nephropathy and neuropathy. However, the effect of intensive therapy on macrovascular disease was less clear. A reduction in all major cardiovascular and peripheral vascular events was observed but this did not reach statistical significance. Patients participating in the study were of relatively young age (under 39 years) which might well have influenced the outcome. At least the DCCT Study found no evidence of increased macrovascular disease with intensive insulin therapy refuting the suggestion that injected insulin itself might predispose to increased atherosclerosis and cardiovascular morbidity. For the moment, the relationship between blood glucose levels and arterial disease remains unproven, but equally so many other likely contributory adverse factors are so dependent on the level of diabetic control, such as hyperlipidaemia, platelet adhesiveness and fibrinogen levels, that it still makes prudent practice to ensure as good a glycaemic control as possible for both IDDM and NIDDM. It is to be hoped that the UK Prospective Diabetes Study[8] involving study of a number of differing treatment regimens for NIDDM over many years and now drawing to its concluding stages may provide some further light on this area.

Another aspect concerning arterial risk in diabetes relates to observed alteration in gender susceptibility. Although both males and females with diabetes carry increased risk of arterial disease, the susceptibility is particularly so for the female, whose normal pre-menopausal advantage and protection from coronary heart disease is lost in the presence of diabetes. Once more the explanation may be complex with interaction between obesity issues and hormonal changes[9]. Unfavourable fat distribution, particularly central adiposity, sometimes described as android obesity can be linked with increased androgenecity of underlying hormonal levels. In particular sex hormone binding globulin (SHBG) is inversely related to overall and upper body adiposity, and in turn associates with an atherogenic pattern of cardiovascular risk factors, including free testosterone levels, increased triglycerides and reduced HDL cholesterol. These observations raise the question as to whether hormone replacement therapy (HRT) has benefit to offer the post-menopausal diabetic lady. There has been some report that oestrogen can provide cardio-protective benefits for diabetic women, while at the same time it would seem as though the oestrogen component of HRT has no significant adverse effect on diabetic control. Progestogen may attenuate the benefit by a small adverse effect on insulin mediated glucose uptake but the effects seem small and unlikely to cancel potential benefits of oestrogen therapy on the cardiovascular circulation.

Much of the increased prevalence of arterial disease with diabetes can be strongly related to the presence of cardiovascular risk factors. Each factor confers its own increased risk, but equally the more factors that are interactive the greater the risk becomes. The accumulative effect of multiple risk factors on the cardiovascular system is well known for the non-diabetic population, and it would seem as though the presence of diabetes at least doubles the risk for each combination of factors be it single or multiple. Risk factors themselves simply indicate increased likelihood of cardiovascular disease, and are not necessarily causal. If risk factors are simply a reflection of increased susceptibility, it could be argued that risk factor intervention would have minimal benefit. However, the argument that risk factors actively contribute to the process of premature arterial disease is substantial, and gradually evidence that improved outcome results from modifying and eliminating adverse risk factors is emerging. Present understanding is that risk factors should be actively identified and individually addressed on the premiss that they are significant and potentially reversible contributors to increased cardiovascular morbidity and mortality.

HYPERTENSION

The combination of raised blood pressure and diabetes is a serious situation, posing increased predisposition to cardiovascular morbidity and mortality[10]. The relationship between hypertension and diabetes has been extensively studied and, although at times the specific relationship between the two has been unclear, there now seems little doubt that hypertension does occur more commonly with diabetes, that its presence does confer greater prospect of complications developing and that it should thereby be taken as seriously as glycaemic control when planning appropriate treatment strategies. In a few rare cases the combination of hypertension and diabetes will draw attention to other underlying endocrine disorders such as acromegaly or Cushing's disorder, but usually the clinical features of such will provide sufficient suspicion of diagnosis to lead to appropriate investigation. In most instances, no such obvious disorder is identified. In early years of insulin-dependent diabetes blood pressure levels may not be detectably abnormal, but from late adolescence onwards a degree of elevation, sometimes known as micro-hypertension, may be observed, and when associated with microalbuminuria[11] a complex interaction can ensue. Blood pressure inevitably rises with more advanced nephropathy, but even in the absence of detectable renal abnormality, high blood pressure does become more evident with longer duration of insulin-dependent diabetes. Up to 20% of IDDM patients with diabetes duration in excess of 15 years may have diastolic blood pressure levels above 100 mmHg compared with 11.5% of an aged matched population. With non-insulin-dependent diabetes, the incidence is even greater. In the UK prospective multi-centre study 40% of males and 53% of females recorded blood pressure levels in excess of 160/95.

Whatever the incidence of hypertension, the effect on mortality and morbidity seems beyond dispute. The presence of hypertension in diabetes is associated with reduced survival, the predominant cause of death being myocardial infarction in 40% of cases. Long-term longitudinal studies show a substantial increase in mortality in the presence of both hypertension and diabetes. Furthermore, the individual increased risk of both hypertension and diabetes is not just simply doubled when the two occur together, but the combination increases the risk exponentially with greatest risk for young adults, especially women.

The effect of hypertension on the development of microvascular complications seems reasonably established in that hypertension will accelerate decline in established nephropathy, eventually contributing to end stage renal failure, as well as eye disorders such as exudative retinopathy and retinal vein thrombosis. The effect of hypertension on large vessel disease is more debatable for, to some extent, hypertension may be a secondary reflection of disordered blood vessels with loss of arterial elasticity. The primary role of hypertension leading to large vessel problems, is unclear. None the less, lowering of elevated blood pressure is likely to be associated with reduction in cerebral haemorrhagic events, lessening of cardiac failure and improvement in peripheral arterial blood flow.

The cause of raised blood pressure in diabetes is equally complex but almost certainly includes an essential genetic component and variable interaction with disturbance of the metabolic state including altered vascular reactivity, sodium retention and possibly a consequence of hyperinsulinism in the insulin-resistant state. Considerable attention has been paid to the potential causative role of hyperinsulinism leading to hypertension, but the conclusion is still uncertain. It is unlikely to be a simple link for in cases of spontaneous hyperinsulinism, such as seen with insulinoma, hypertension is not a usual feature.

Treatment of hypertension is important and should be properly screened, assessed and treated as carefully as the blood sugar. Inevitably there are specific therapeutic considerations. Initial management of the hypertensive diabetic should include advice on lifestyle, the patient being encouraged to reduce excessive weight, to modify diet by reducing sodium and saturated fat intake and to limit alcohol consumption. Pharmacological treatment is complex, often confusing and frequently complicating. On the one hand hypotensive drugs are prescribed in an endeavour to reduce vascular risk, while on the other hand many drugs carry particular problems for the diabetic patient. The relationship between hypotensive drugs and glucose intolerance has been reviewed[12].

For instance, beta blockers can have an inhibiting effect on insulin secretion which may unmask latent maturity onset diabetes or aggravate control in a known NIDDM. With insulin-dependent diabetes beta blockers can affect hypoglycaemic awareness and impair recovery from such. Calcium channel blocking agents appear to have no sustained effect on glucose tolerance at conventional dosage but can give rise to side effects including flushing and orthostatic hypotension. In recent years ACE inhibitors have found a special role in the treatment of hypertension in diabetes, particularly with nephropathy and also left ventricular dysfunction. However, care needs to be taken in patients with ischaemic renal disease or significant aortic outflow obstruction. Prolonged usage of potassium losing diuretics, particularly thiazides, can result in deterioration of glucose tolerance, although the effect is relatively small when these drugs are used at low dosage.

HYPERLIPIDAEMIA

It is not always recognized that disorder of lipid metabolism is as much part of the process of diabetes mellitus as is abnormality of carbohydrate metabolism. Indeed, disturbance of circulating lipid profiles may be the predominant abnormality with disturbed metabolism in diabetes[13]. So often with NIDDM venous samples are reported as showing significant lipaemia while the blood sugar itself may not be that high. It is also difficult to classify lipid abnormalities into convenient labelled categories, for it is possible for individual patients to exhibit all variations on a theme of hyperlipidaemia cascading through several different types according to the degree of disruption of diabetes control. All patients with diabetes have the potential to develop abnormal lipid profiles, and at any one time as many as 25% of patients attending a diabetes clinic will demonstrate lipid abnormality. In many of these the abnormality is related to poor control of diabetes, i.e. a likely secondary consequence, but in many others the level of diabetic control may be good, suggesting that hyperlipidaemia may be an independent contributory risk factor.

Although patterns may differ between IDDM and NIDDM, a common basis for disturbed lipid metabolism can still be identified. Insulin deficiency is still an essential component, be it absolute (IDDM) or relative (insulin resistance/NIDDM)[14]. The consequence of insulin deficiency or that of insulin resistance is much the same. Hypertriglyceridaemia predominates as insulin lack leads to reduced lipoprotein lipase activity, and thereby decreased clearance of circulating triglycerides and low HDL levels. Furthermore, increased lipolysis occurs in adipose tissue and an increase of free fatty acids is delivered to the liver, with resultant fatty change. It should be recognized that total cholesterol is an independent variable of diabetes but the LDL fraction may be significantly affected by such. As a result total cholesterol levels with diabetes are likely to reflect the pattern in the population at large with a contributory cardiovascular risk according to the precise level. However, with diabetes it is important to be aware that for a given level of total cholesterol the unfavourable LDL sub-fraction may be a much lower percentage than in non-diabetes and should be specifically measured. Even if the total cholesterol level is not that high, a low LDL sub-fraction of the order of 10% in the presence of diabetes would be an indication for more active therapeutic intervention.

Protocols for the management of diabetes now include recommendations on measurement of lipids, although the detail concerning when to treat is more variable and uncertain. With IDDM total cholesterol and LDL sub-fraction should be known from early adulthood, say after 25 years of age. For NIDDM, where hypertriglyceridaemia can predominate, a full lipid profile including sub-fractions should be done at diagnosis and at annual review.

When hyperlipidaemia is found, attention should be paid to optimizing diabetic control in the first instance. Particular emphasis should be placed on diet[15], aiming towards weight loss when appropriate, reduction in total fat intake to about 30% of total energy intake, and adjustment of fat balance towards more polyunsaturated/monounsaturated oils. Indeed, the relatively high fat consumption of earlier diabetic diets, when absolute carbohydrate restriction was imposed, could well have contributed to the observed increased prevalence of atherosclerosis in diabetes, and it is to be hoped that the change towards greater consumption of unrefined starch based carbohydrate and consequent lessening of total fat consumption will prove beneficial in this respect. Protocols for drug intervention with lipid lowering agents are still being formulated, but in general hyperlipidaemia with diabetes poses a double risk factor such that the situation should be tackled that much more actively than when diabetes is not present. A total cholesterol greater than 7.3 mmol/l increases coronary heart disease risk five-fold compared with a total cholesterol level of less than 5.5 mmol/l. Precise targets are difficult to give for the diabetic population as a whole, and do need to be set sensibly at an individual level. The gold standard for total cholesterol is 5.2 mmol/l and should be targeted if any cardiovascular event has occurred. In the absence of overt cardiovascular disease the total cholesterol in patients with diabetes should be below 5.5 mmol/l with at least 20% HDL fraction. Levels above these targets despite dietary adjustment should merit consideration of drug treatment. Hypertriglyceridaemia, much more susceptible to fluctuations in diabetic control, has its own independent cardiovascular risk effect and if abnormality is sustained despite optimization of diabetic control and dietary adherence, drug therapy should again be reviewed.

A variety of drugs is available for lowering abnormal lipid levels and the choice of drug requires consideration of the specific profile of the hyperlipidaemia that has been identified. With mixed hyperlipidaemia, raised triglycerides and raised cholesterol, fibrate therapy would be the first of choice, and indeed there is evidence that improvement of hyperlipidaemia with fibrate therapy can in turn improve diabetic control, particularly in those with insulin resistance. Where the lipid abnormality is primarily that of elevated cholesterol, HMG CoA reductase inhibitors (statins) are helpful. With increasing experience of statin usage, no adverse effect on diabetes has been observed, and the possibility that these drugs have the potential to reverse some of the earlier stages of atherosclerotic development, may make them particularly attractive for the diabetic patient with hyperlipidaemia. Acipimox is somewhat better tolerated than nicotinic acid derivatives and would be appropriate for isolated hyper-triglyceridaemia.

OBESITY

In the past it has been thought that obesity is not necessarily associated with increased cardiovascular risk, unless additional factors such as hypertension or diabetes are present. More recently, recognition that differing distribution of body fat may be relevant has led to awareness that unfavourable fat distribution may be an independent indicator of circulatory risk. Central adiposity, with increased underlying visceral fat and sometimes known as android obesity, is associated with increased predisposition to premature circulatory disorder. Android distribution of fat or 'apple shape' contrasts with gynoid adiposity or 'pear shape' where fat is largely concentrated on the hips, buttocks and thighs. With gynoid obesity cardiovascular complications are relatively less common. The waist–hip circumference ratio (WHR) can, therefore, be a useful indicator of risk, with a WHR greater than 0.9 pointing to the potential of significant cardiovascular problems ahead.

With diabetes, the relationship between body weight and obesity becomes quite complex. Insulin deficiency itself is associated with reduction in body fat and overall weight loss, while excessive insulin administration is associated frequently with unacceptable weight gain. Central obesity in diabetes, sometimes known as diabesity, forms part of the spectrum of the insulin resistant (Reaven's) syndrome, interacting with other cardiovascular risk factors already discussed.

The cause of obesity in diabetes, as with every risk factor so far discussed, is multifactorial. Undoubtedly there is a genetic basis, with some patients more predisposed than others on the basis of the genes they have inherited. Differing metabolisms may have some basis on differing inherited traits. Having said that, there is no doubt that lifestyle factors can have an equal if not greater contribution to the development of obesity and it is these that are potentially reversible.

Treatment strategies should, therefore, be directed to improving such lifestyle factors by proper dietary advice, preferably under the guidance of a dietitian, with sensible and appropriate weight reduction as required.

Along with diet, a reasonable exercise programme should be advised in order to maintain an adequate metabolic rate which otherwise simply diminishes as calorie consumption is reduced. Despite the best of intentions with diet and exercise, long-term results are disappointing. Initial enthusiasm and motivation may well meet with success, but so often the situation is difficult to sustain and weight is slowly regained.

Pharmacological intervention for obesity requires much more careful consideration and selective usage under specialist supervision. D-Flen-fluramine, which appears to alter central serotonin concentrations, can result in prompt reduction in blood sugar levels and later significant weight loss but considerable determination is required to maintain the achieved benefits once the recommended three-month treatment period has taken place and drug treatment has been withdrawn. Calculation of the body mass index (BMI) takes into account the ratio of weight to height, and allows an index of cardiovascular risk to be determined. For instance, a desirable BMI would be between 20.0 and 25.0, but once the BMI rises above 30.0 mortality risk increases substantially, with the term morbid obesity being used once the BMI is in excess of 40.

CIGARETTE SMOKING

Of all the risk factors, cigarette smoking[16] should be the one that is most readily reversible but in practice is less easily achieved. Indeed, the benefits of stopping smoking in diabetes may exceed other therapeutic measures for associated hypertension and hyperlipidaemia. Cigarette smoking in diabetes has been linked with increased risk of developing microangiopathic complications, such as nephropathy and retinopathy, but the greatest adverse affect, is on vascular morbidity and mortality. In a large cross-sectional review[17] of a busy diabetic clinic, the author observed a significant reduction in male smokers with diabetes compared with a control non-diabetic group due to premature death. Cigarette smoking in combination with diabetes significantly reduces the prospects of men reaching pensionable age. Although the situation was less clear with women with diabetes, because of the then smaller numbers who smoked, it is probable that, given the increase susceptibility to coronary heart disease of the diabetic woman, the risk may be even greater. It would seem as though cigarette smoking doubles the risk of premature mortality in insulin-dependent diabetes, and while the risk with NIDDM is more complex because of the interaction with multiple risk factors, cigarette smoking continues to be a strong and separate predictor of risk in its own right.

Cerebrovascular episodes and coronary heart events occur more frequently and with greater severity in diabetic people who smoke.

However, it is with peripheral arterial disease of the legs where this effect is most evident, with the most severe problems of such arising from this deadly combination. Intermittent claudication of the leg, ulceration of the foot and lower limb amputation are all strongly associated with a combination of cigarette smoking and diabetes. Unfortunately advanced end stage peripheral vascular disease reaches a point where stopping smoking makes little difference to eventual outcome. It is to be regretted how often good intentions to stop smoking are expressed when serious consequences develop, but too late for benefit to follow. None the less, improvement in peripheral blood flow can be demonstrated in those with arterial insufficiency of the leg, at an earlier stage of the process before the limb becomes threatened irretrievably by progressive ischaemia. Cigarette smoking not only exerts a detrimental effect on the circulation, but also adversely influences diabetic control, partly as a consequence of the direct patho-pharmacological effects of smoking, but also from associated other poor aspects of lifestyle. People with diabetes may not smoke any more than the normal population, and the reasons for smoking may be similar, but if an effective means could be found to discourage cigarette smoking in those with diabetes before severe vascular problems develop, the dividend could be considerable.

HEART DISEASE

The heart in diabetes is affected in different ways[18], with variable contribution from myocardial dysfunction, autonomic neuropathy and ischaemic heart disease. The latter, as a consequence of the coronary occlusive process, contributes to the substantial morbidity and mortality that arises from large vessel disease in diabetes. As death from end stage renal failure in insulin-dependent diabetes diminishes, death from coronary heart disease rises. For NIDDM mortality from coronary disease is even greater and overall, for those deaths recorded in association with diabetes, at least 50% are probably and primarily due to coronary disease. The various clinical expressions of coronary disease, angina, acute myocardial infarction and heart failure, all occur more commonly with diabetes, often presenting at an earlier age and with greater severity. Epidemiological observations indicate geographical variation in the frequency of clinical coronary disorder, being as low as 6% prevalence in Japan, in contrast to the much higher proportion in the Western world. As earlier discussed, this would suggest an environmental lifestyle effect, probably of a dietary nature, for the apparent protection is lost when Western lifestyle is adopted. The earlier presentation of coronary disease in IDDM is often evident by the fourth decade and not infrequently significant coronary disease may present at an even younger age, including ladies well before the menopause. With NIDDM some evidence of underlying coronary disorder, be it clinical or electrocardiographic, is frequently present at diagnosis, often in association with detectable cerebrovascular and peripheral arterial disease of the legs as well. All coronary manifestations occur more frequently, and to greater severity, while the trend towards a decline in the coronary mortality rate of the population at large is not as yet so clearly evident for diabetes.

ANGINA

The classical description of exertional constricting central chest tightness may not always be obtained, despite severe underlying coronary disease. Symptoms described may be much more subtle and atypical, including simple fatigue, which may obscure accurate diagnosis. This is particularly so when the patient is young and female, and the diagnosis does not seem probable. However, unusual chest symptoms, particularly with an exertional component, must be taken seriously, for it is known that 'silent' (asymptomatic) ischaemia frequently occurs, and indeed clinically evident angina is likely to represent the tip of the iceberg phenomenon.

When angina is suspected, or as part of a review screening protocol for asymptomatic patients, an electrocardiograph may be helpful. ST segment or T wave abnormalities may be detected suggesting underlying ischaemia, and not infrequently signs of previously unsuspected old myocardial infarction may be present. Further abnormality may be elicited with treadmill exercise ECG investigation, and positive tests may be found in up to 25% of NIDDM patients without symptoms and also in a significant proportion of established IDDM with duration of diabetes longer than 15 years. Such is the extent of potential silent coronary disease that many could be identified by exercise testing, the need and implications of investigating for asymptomatic coronary disease have been debated[19]. At the moment there is no clear evidence that those without symptoms but with positive exercise ECGs are any the better managed for that knowledge, and it is doubtful whether present resources could meet the potential demand of further investigation including angiography, and its treatment consequences such as coronary bypass surgery.

Drug therapy for angina in diabetes is similar to that given to non-diabetic anginal sufferers, but some care needs to be taken. This is particularly so with use of beta blockers, which can modify hypoglycaemic awareness in the IDDM patient and also exert a moderate deleterious affect on glucose and lipid metabolism in the NIDDM. In the presence of peripheral arterial disease, claudication and cold feet can be aggravated. Beta blockers should not necessarily be regarded as contraindicated for in certain individuals they may prove useful in the control of angina, but care is needed to select patients appropriately with these considerations in mind. Calcium channel blockers have no significant clinical effect on diabetes and may be used, while oral nitrates can be particularly helpful. Patients with deteriorating angina, not responding to increasing doses of anti-anginal medication, should be considered for further investigation, initially by treadmill exercise ECG and then coronary arteriography if necessary.

ACUTE MYOCARDIAL INFARCTION

Of all coronary manifestations, much has been reported concerning myocardial infarction in diabetes, emphasizing the increased susceptibility to heart attacks and increased severity of such, with greater frequency of associated problems and higher consequent mortality. As with angina presentation of acute myocardial infarction may be very atypical, often with reduced or absent chest pain, which in turn can lead to failure to establish the correct diagnosis, thereby delaying management and initiation of inappropriate treatment. Patients may present with rather vague chest symptoms, including a feeling of breathlessness rather than pain, and not uncommonly with non-specific symptoms including loss of well-being and tiredness. Deterioration in diabetic glycaemic control may have happened for no obvious explicable reason, and diabetic ketoacidosis may be precipitated by an otherwise silent underlying myocardial infarction. These considerations have important implications for the early management of acute myocardial infarction and so a high index of suspicion must be maintained with diabetes presenting acutely with non-specific symptoms or unexplained loss of control.

Increased risk of myocardial infarction with diabetes is a reflection of the accelerated and more severe atherosclerotic occlusive disease process of the coronary arteries. Larger infarct size, particularly full thickness, is observed and complications of myocardial infarction including arrhythmia, conduction disorder and cardiogenic shock occur more commonly. As a result mortality with acute myocardial infarction is significantly worse in diabetes, with approximately two-fold increased mortality risk in men, and three-fold in women. Immediate mortality from myocardial infarction in diabetes is as high as 34% compared with about 18% when diabetes is not present, while at 6 months up to 50% mortality has been reported. This increased mortality is likely to reflect the greater severity of underlying coronary disease and the fact that more complications occur during the acute stages. However, the predominant reason for poor outcome is that of myocardial pump failure.

Hyperglycaemia, with blood sugar in excess of 11 mmol/l, is commonly found in cases of acute myocardial infarction presenting to coronary care units[20], and is often attributed to 'stress' hyperglycaemia, such that in years past blood sugar elevation has been regarded similar to that of rise in cardiac enzymes. The precise nature of stress hyperglycaemia is debated but in many instances a presumed susceptibility to diabetes is present, which is unmasked at times of particular stress. In others, observed hyperglycaemia can be a genuine indication of preceding, unsuspected diabetes. Whatever its nature, hyperglycaemia is associated with a more adverse outcome in proportion to the level of blood sugar. Hyperglycaemia associates with other adverse metabolic disturbance, including increased release of free fatty acids, suppression of insulin secretion, and rise in catabolic hormones, which in turn may aggravate tendency to arrhythmias and impair myocardial contractility, leading to greater severity of cardiac failure.

Coronary care unit management of acute myocardial infarction complicating diabetes requires particular skilled management and guidelines for glycaemic control should be made available. All patients should have an initial blood sugar estimation on admission to the coronary care unit. Levels above 11 mmol/l should be checked 1 hour later. Sugars remaining persistently elevated should be actively treated. In most cases, either IDDM or NIDDM, low dose intravenous insulin infusion according to written protocols is the preferred method of management. Cardiac complications arising in NIDDM probably do so from the disturbed metabolic state, but those on oral agents may do less well than those treated by insulin. In practical terms, for those where the blood sugar rapidly falls back to single figures, tablets may be continued or indeed temporarily withdrawn, while for those whose sugars remain elevated intravenous insulin remains the preferred therapy of choice. During convalescence, when the stress effect on diabetes has settled, review of treatment and return to oral agents can be made.

Other therapeutic aspects in the management of myocardial infarction should follow general principles and guidelines. It is worth commenting that the use of angiotensin-converting enzyme inhibitors (ACE inhibitors) may have a special beneficial role with diabetes. It is now favoured practice to introduce an ACE inhibitor at an early stage of acute myocardial infarction, particularly full thickness anterior and for those considered at risk of left ventricular dysfunction. By its nature those with diabetes are more likely to be in this category, such that early usage of ACE inhibitors should have a significant impact on outcome, particularly towards lessening of cardiac failure and reduction in subsequent mortality. Diabetic patients suffering acute myocardial infarction may require a longer stay in hospital before discharge home. Treatment on discharge should include low dose aspirin therapy and in all probability an ACE inhibitor as well. At follow-up review, other potential contributory risk factors should be addressed and duly dealt with as needed. Consideration of further cardiac investigation should follow the same criteria as for non-diabetes, and the presence of diabetes should not be regarded as a specific contraindication. It should be recognized that coronary arteriography is likely to show more severe changes involving all three main vessels and of a more diffuse and distal nature. The latter does create greater technical difficulty for successful coronary bypass grafting, but in many instances lesions may be only proximal, and thereby amenable to either angioplasty or bypass surgery. Each case deserves consideration on an individual basis.

CARDIAC FAILURE

Primary myocardial failure in diabetes is a major determinant of cardiac morbidity and mortality. The risk of cardiac failure for men with IDDM increases two-fold and for women five-fold, once more identifying the greater adverse effect of diabetes in the female. Similarly, with NIDDM increased predisposition to angina and myocardial infarction is accompanied by greater severity of heart failure. Coronary artery disease significantly contributes to the development of heart failure either acutely with myocardial infarction or more insidiously in association with increasing angina. In many cases, underlying myocardial ischaemia remains undetected, until cardiac failure presents. The diabetic myocardium may show diffuse fibrotic changes as a consequence of ischaemia, and possible preceding, subclinical microinfarcts. The aetiology of heart failure in diabetes is complex. Apart from the clear effect of coronary disease, myocardial function may be impaired directly by adverse metabolic changes, such as glycoprotein deposition, and possibly in some instances by the development of microangiopathy. As a result of such observations the term diabetic cardiomyopathy[21] has been introduced, when primary myocardial disturbance is often out of proportion to the severity of the coronary disease. The presence of obesity, hypertension and nephropathy contribute their own aggravating influence on the already compromised myocardium, and thereby accelerate decline in cardiac function.

Acute left ventricular failure is a common consequence of acute myocardial infarction in diabetes, often severe because of the greater magnitude of the coronary event. The degree of left ventricular dysfunction is the major determinant of outcome following myocardial infarction and is responsible for the greater case fatality observed with diabetes, both in the immediate post-myocardial infarction period and over subsequent months.

In contrast, development of heart failure may be more insidious presenting without history of angina or infarction. Slowly developing exertional breathlessness can sometimes be difficult to distinguish from angina, when central chest tightness may be felt more as difficulty in breathing than as pain as such. Exertional breathlessness, particularly on walking up an incline or upstairs and on lying flat in bed at night, should raise suspicion of underlying left ventricular failure. Signs on physical examination may be very deceptive initially with no clinical evidence of cardiac enlargement, while added chest sounds may be minimal or even absent. Similarly, the chest X-ray may prove unhelpful for the stiffer diabetic myocardium reduces cardiac enlargement, giving rise to apparent normal cardiac size. Electrocardiography may show presence of previously unsuspected old myocardial infarction but often no clear abnormality is evident. Echo cardiography can be helpful in revealing poor left ventricular contractility, reduced end diastolic ejection fraction, and overall global restriction of myocardial function.

With the passage of time, heart failure becomes more manifest, often associated with relapsing bouts of acute left ventricular failure, leading to recurrent hospital admission with severe distressing breathlessness. With prompt intravenous diuretic therapy it is remarkable how often quick return to apparent normality can be achieved once fluid overload has been relieved. With such admissions it is unusual to find significant ECG or cardiac enzyme changes. The episode simply reflects the increasing incapacity of the diabetic myocardium to cope with maintaining a normal cardiac output and circulation, illustrating the fine and precarious balance of the situation. Left ventricular dysfunction predominates during the early stages of chronic failure in diabetes, but eventually congestive cardiac failure ensues with added right heart features, particularly oedema of the legs, becoming increasingly apparent.

Heart failure is worsened by poor diabetic control, and in turn is aggravated at the time of acute episodes of hyperglycaemia, thus creating a vicious circle. It is, therefore, important to ensure good control of diabetes both when the heart failure is stable and when acute exacerbations occur. Loop diuretics have a first line role in the management of heart failure, either intravenously for acute episodes or as maintenance therapy once the situation is stabilized. Continuation of maintenance diuretics may be more finely balanced with diabetes, for withdrawal of diuretic, be it advised or otherwise, can lead to abrupt onset of left ventricular failure. The most significant development in the treatment of heart failure with diabetes has been the introduction of ACE inhibitor therapy which does seem to have a special role in diabetes. Indeed, the very usage of ACE inhibitor therapy has probably altered the natural history of heart failure, leading to longer survival and the reason why patients with chronic heart failure, interrupted by episodes of acute LVF, survive and struggle on, whereas previously they would not have done so. Most diabetic patients with heart failure can be treated successfully with ACE inhibitor therapy, but the commencement of treatment should follow usual precautions with the first administration, namely starting with a small test dose under supine conditions, taking specific care to exclude patients with likely aortic outflow obstruction (by echo cardiography if necessary) or renal ischaemia. Patients who have been treated with diuretics for sometime prior to initiation of ACE inhibitor therapy, should have the first dose administered under hospital supervision, usually as a day case. Potassium levels should be monitored, and usually the ACE inhibitor effect is sufficient to offset the potassium losing effect of loop diuretics. The potassium sparing diuretics can be particularly prone to cause hyperkalaemia in diabetes and should be avoided when an ACE inhibitor is introduced. As heart failure progresses and resultant increasing doses of diuretics are used, the electrolyte balance becomes even more difficult to maintain. Fluid accumulation in extravascular tissues increases while the intravascular compartment becomes increasingly hypovolaemic. Addition of a thiazide to existing loop diuretic therapy can often enhance diuresis and improve cardiac failure, but in due course these electrolyte difficulties become increasingly difficult to manage.

Revascularization of the myocardium offers little benefit to the patient with cardiac failure and so coronary bypass surgery is unlikely to be helpful in this situation. Cardiac transplantation may be considered for severe end stage diabetic heart failure, and indeed a number of diabetic cases have received heart transplants. However, the presence of diabetes poses special difficulties, and the presence of other long-term complications seriously affects outcome, such that cardiac transplantation is not generally regarded as a treatment option available for the diabetic patient.

CEREBROVASCULAR DISEASE

The diffuse effect of diabetes on the circulation is also manifest by a greatly increased cerebrovascular disease. Carotid arteries show more severe changes and multiple stenotic lesions are often present. The diffuse nature of the atherosclerosis means that a severe narrowing or occlusion of a vessel will have a greater adverse affect, as collateral blood supply is likely to be poor as well. Atherosclerosis of the great vessels proceeds, usually in parallel with coronary and peripheral arterial disease, by endothelial plaque formation and progressive occlusion. Carotid artery bruits are frequently detected before clinical symptoms develop.

The clinical consequences of disturbed posterior circulation include vertebrobasilar insufficiency and incoordination of the limbs. A feeling of dizziness, or sudden blackouts, provoked by extension or rotation of the neck, leads to diagnosis of vertebrobasilar insufficiency, often associated with unsteadiness of gait and other cerebellar features. The most common early manifestation of carotid artery disease is that of a transient ischaemic attack (TIA), with sudden development of weakness or sensory change in contralateral limbs, or alternatively temporary disruption to vision in one eye (amaurosis fugax). These episodes are likely to be embolic, with clots arising from plaques within the carotid arteries. In many instances the attack is of a temporary nature with minimal or no residual neurological disabilities, but it provides warning of the potential severe stroke that could be ahead. Total occlusion of a single carotid artery does not necessarily result in a completed stroke if collateral blood supply is still adequate, but with diabetes the risk of a major cerebrovascular episode[22] with permanent neurological deficit is that much greater, rather similar observations to that seen with acute myocardial infarction. For instance, when compared with those without diabetes, a stroke in a diabetic patient is associated with a greater degree of neurological disability, a greater immediate case fatality, a worse long-term prognosis and a greater risk of a further episode. As with myocardial infarction, a high proportion of all stroke cases, in some reports up to 25%, may have an elevated blood sugar on admission. A number of these will have preceding undiagnosed diabetes, possibly of the order of 8%, while in others the elevated blood sugar reflects stress hyperglycaemia. Even if it is shown that the haemoglobin A1C is normal, thereby excluding significant preceding diabetes, stress hyperglycaemia still appears to be associated with more unfavourable outcome. Good control of blood sugar following an acute cerebrovascular episode is likely to be particularly important in determining the eventual outcome.

A more insidious cerebral vascular development is that of dementia, with atherosclerosis leading to progressive reduction in cerebral blood flow, often further aggravated by the occurrence of multiple infarcts. Some of these result from carotid artery emboli and in such cases a history of TIAs may be obtained. In others, multiple infarcts may result from diffuse disease of small vessels within the brain causing patchy ischaemia and local thrombosis. Development of multi-infarct dementia is characterized by initial impairment of higher cerebral function, particularly concentration and memory, and later by more severe disturbance of mood, behaviour and global cerebral activity.

In terms of investigation, the detection of a carotid artery bruit or the occurrence of a TIA requires initial assessment by Doppler ultrasound studies, to demonstrate the degree of occlusive disorder and thereby determine what further needs to be done. The severity of plaque formation can usually be ascertained by this procedure and serve as a guide to the most appropriate therapy. Internal carotid artery diameter occlusion of greater than 80% requires consideration of further investigation with a view to possible surgery. Lesser occlusion may be managed medically if previous treatment with aspirin has not been given. The occurrence of further TIA while on aspirin therapy requires further investigation. Such cases need carotid angiography, proceeding to endartarectomy where necessary. For those managed conservatively, low dose aspirin therapy is the single most important treatment to offer. The level of blood sugar also has important effects on cerebrovascular blood flow and so it is important to ensure as good a control of diabetes as is possible. Blood pressure also requires special attention as hypertension is associated with increased cerebrovascular risk. Characteristically, in diabetic patients with large vessel disease, the blood pressure exhibits systolic but not necessarily diastolic elevation, i.e. a wide pulse pressure. The cause and effects of such systolic elevation are debated, and in part it is due to a greater rigidity and loss of elasticity of vessels rather than true hypertension. Furthermore, undue lowering of blood pressure runs the risk of critical reduction in cerebral blood flow and aggravation of underlying cerebrovascular disease. In general, elevated diastolic blood pressure levels, e.g. above 95–100 mmHg, require consideration of therapeutic intervention, while treatment of systolic hypertension, particularly in diabetes, is a much more uncertain issue. That systolic hypertension is associated with increased cardiovascular morbidity and mortality is not doubted, but until the debate as to whether it is simply an indicator of underlying vascular disease or a risk factor in its own right, careful thought should be given before introducing potent drug therapy.

PERIPHERAL ARTERIAL DISEASE OF THE LEGS

To complete the major triad of large vessel disease in diabetes, peripheral arterial disease of the lower limb gives rise to a considerable number of clinical and management issues[23]. The ischaemic leg so often appears to be the prerogative of the diabetic patient, and so often ends in the individual tragedy of required amputation. Furthermore, admissions due to diabetic foot problems, as a consequence of impaired circulation, absorb a considerable and disproportionate amount of hospital bed occupancy. The costs of amputation are substantial, and there is presently no other area of diabetes practice that has the opportunity for greater long-term health gain if more investment of resources were to be made to prevent the terrible consequences of large vessel disease in the leg.

The diabetic foot, discussed in detail in Chapter 7, comprises several aspects contributing to risk, including the combination of neuropathy, trauma, infection and arterial insufficiency. These factors, present to varying degree in the individual, combine to pose major risk of serious foot problems. To some extent the circulatory disorder of the leg in diabetes is different to that in the non-diabetic. Diffuse atherosclerotic changes can be observed, but equally patchy involvement is not uncommon and in particular more distal involvement can be a specific feature.

This variability of involvement of the peripheral arteries to the leg, gives rise to different patterns of clinical presentation. Paradoxically, more distal involvement of large vessels is often associated with less exercise induced symptoms such as claudication, such that the first manifestation of circulatory insufficiency in the diabetic patient is often ulceration of the foot or gangrenous change of the toe. Prior to such, the patient may have been unaware that the circulation to the leg was impaired. The development of a foot ulcer, commonly through inadvertent and unsuspected trauma, or the sudden appearance of a gangrenous toe quickly draws attention to the serious underlying ischaemic problem. The truly ischaemic foot is cold, red with dependency and pale on elevation, with pulses weak or indeed absent. Careful palpation for pedal pulses remains an important part of examination of the risk foot in diabetes.

Large vessel disease is almost certainly the major contributory cause of circulatory problems in the diabetic foot, and the issue of whether significant microangiopathy can be a significant factor is still debated. It is possible that functional disturbance of the micro circulation may lead to reduced nutrient supply to subcutaneous tissues, impaired healing and possibly reduced oxygen supply. Diffuse small vessel disease should not be presumed for such a view can serve as a deterrent for consideration of revascularization to the foot, when successful arterial bypass surgery with an adequate distal vascular anastomosis might still be quite feasible.

Diabetic foot ulceration or detection of potentially critical ischaemic change of the foot requires investigation. Doppler ultrasound investigation, a non-invasive procedure, should be done initially, with simultaneous measurement of arterial pressures at different levels along the lower limb. This technique can identify the particular arterial segments that are most involved by atherosclerotic change and can provide guidance as to whether successful revascularization of the leg can be contemplated. One difficulty may arise when medial calcinosis is present in tibial vessels, giving rise to artificially high detected pressures. Under such circumstances careful clinical consideration, particularly taking into account the quality of foot pulses, becomes most important. Doppler ultrasound studies may permit direct progression to vascular surgery, but angiography is often needed to ensure the best chance of success with arterial reconstruction. Undoubtedly, the availability of skilled and experienced vascular surgery offers the most immediate and best opportunity for reducing the need for amputation in diabetes, which still remains distressingly high.

In the long term it is to be hoped that preventive measures will reduce the numbers of patients with diabetes progressing to such serious circulatory consequences, which not only threaten loss of limb and mobility, but also associate with significant mortality risk as well. Until the precise metabolic relationship in the development of atherosclerosis in diabetes is elucidated, large vessel disease is likely to continue as a major and demanding clinical problem. As earlier discussed, attention to risk factors could well have a major impact. Cigarette smoking can increase the prospect of serious peripheral arterial disease of the leg by as much as 50-fold, while cessation of smoking may improve peripheral blood flow by as much as 50% within 6 months. A similar relationship to hypertension can be observed, with improved blood supply to the leg following effective control of blood pressure.

CONCLUSION

Large vessel disease contributes significantly to premature morbidity and mortality in diabetes. Already known to be a substantial problem with non-insulin-dependent diabetes, awareness of its importance with insulin-dependent diabetes becomes increasingly apparent as microvascular complications become more effectively contained. Large vessel disease in diabetes is probably the most important clinical challenge ahead, and the outstanding complication to be addressed. The present tragedy is that so often major circulatory disorder develops during a long and silent period such that, when clinically evident, the consequences are already severe, critical and potentially life threatening. It is a tragedy that first clinical awareness of such problems may be an extensive myocardial infarction, refractory cardiac failure, a major cerebrovascular catastrophe or a gangrenous ulcerated foot. Can such be avoided?

To truly undertake prevention much more understanding of the mechanisms involved in the process of atherosclerosis in diabetes will need to be determined. The underlying causes and mechanisms are still far from clear. Undoubtedly there will be genetic factors, but how are they mediated? What is the relationship to disturbed metabolism and hormone chemistry? What is the relationship to hyperglycaemia when simple glucose intolerance can be associated with advanced arterial risk? Does good control of blood sugar make any difference or should we be striving for as near normal blood sugar levels as possible? Can good control of diabetes be commenced as early as possible in the process? Yet the clinical presentation is often preceded by a long silent period of metabolic risk, increasing the difficulties of early intervention. NIDDM, in particular, poses a complex situation. The concept of an insulin-resistant syndrome is deliberated and the effects of consequent hyperinsulinism debated. If hyperinsulinism is pathogenic, what is the potential contribution of injected insulin or that stimulated by oral hypoglycaemic therapy? These are questions still to be answered.

Apart from metabolic considerations, acquired or environmental factors do seem very important. Studies relating to nutrition *in utero* and early childhood have drawn attention to a striking potential relationship to future development of arterial disease, but still do not adequately explain acquisition of risk when moving from low to high prevalent areas. It is probable that a fundamental genetic susceptibility interacts with environmental factors, and it is with the latter that the best immediate prospect of successful preventive measures is offered.

Central obesity is a bad indicator of health and associates with risk of diabetes and vascular morbidity. Avoidance and reduction of obesity should be strongly encouraged by dietary measures and appropriate exercise. By a careful and sensible combination of dietary adjustment and increased physical activity weight can be lost, but sustaining the progress is difficult and often disappointing. Maintaining support and motivation is an important part of management in this respect. Cardiovascular risk factors significantly contribute to the development of arterial problems in diabetes, and risk factor assessment, including hypertension, hyperlipidaemia and cigarette consumption, should be an important part of any guidelines being followed for the management of diabetes.

The sooner evidence of developing large vessel disease is detected, the earlier effective interventional therapy can be initiated. A high degree of suspicion should be held for those at potential risk, especially those with bad family histories of diabetes and associated vascular disease. Once the presence of diabetes is known, review protocols should include essential screening guidelines for the early detection of large vessel disorder. Reduction and indeed prevention of large vessel arterial disease with diabetes still poses considerable difficulties in the present management of patients with diabetes[24], but, by these means of early detection and risk factor intervention, there is reasonable optimism that dividends can be obtained and the more serious consequences lessened. It is to be hoped that the recent considerable advances in the management of microvascular disease of diabetes will find parallel observation for that of large vessel disease as well.

REFERENCES

1 Steiner G. Atherosclerosis, the major complication of diabetes. In: Vranic M, Hollenberg CH, Steiner G (eds), *Comparison of Type I and Type II Diabetes.* Plenum Publishing, 1985; 227.

2 Schwartz CJ, Valente AJ, Sprague EA, Kelley JL, Cayatte AJ, Kerbacher JJ, Mowery J, Rozek MM. Pathogenesis of the atherosclerotic lesion: implications for diabetes mellitus. *Diabetes Care* 1992; **15**(9): 1156–67.

3 Klein R. Hyperglycaemia and microvascular and macrovascular disease in diabetes. *Diabetes Care* 1995; **18**: 251–68.

4 Reaven GM. Role of insulin resistance in human disease. Banting Lecture 1988. *Diabetes* 1988; **37**: 1595–607.

5 Stamler J, Vaccaro O, Neaton JD, Wentworth D. Diabetes other risk factors, and 12 year cardiovascular mortality for men screened in the Multiple Risk Factor Intervention Trial. *Diabetes Care* 1993; **16**: 434–44.

6 Barker DJP, Hales CN, Fall CHD, Osmond C, Clark PMS. Non-insulin-dependent diabetes, hypertension and hyperlipidaemia (Syndrome X): Relation to reduced foetal growth. *Diabetologia* 1993; **36**: 62–7.

7 The Diabetes Control and Complications Trial Research Group. The effect of intensive treatment of diabetes on the development and progression of long-term complications in insulin-dependent diabetes mellitus. *N Engl J Med* 1993; **329**: 977–86.

8 United Kingdom Prospective Diabetes Study VIII. Study design, progress and performance. *Diabetologia* 1991; **34**: 877–90.

9 Haffner SM, Katz MS, Dunn JF. Increased upper body and overall adiposity is associated with decreased sex hormone binding globulin in post menopausal women. *Int J Obesity* 1991; **15**: 471–8.

10 Working Group on Hypertension in Diabetes. Statement on hypertension in diabetes: final report. *Arch Intern Med* 1987; **147**: 830–42.

11 Watts GF, Harris R, Shaw KM. The determinants of early nephropathy in insulin-dependent diabetes mellitus. A prospective study based on the urinary excretion of albumin. *Quart J Med* 1991; **288**: 365–78.

12 Furman BL. Drug-induced impairment of glucose tolerance. *Practical Diabetes* 1992; **9**: 19–22.

13 American Diabetes Association: Clinical Practice Recommendations 1995. Detection and management of lipid disorders in diabetes. *Diabetes Care* 1995; **18** (suppl 1): 86–93.

14 Williams B. Insulin resistance: The shape of things to come. *Lancet* 1994; **344**: 521–4.

15 Report of the Cardiovascular Review Group Committee on Medical Aspects of Food Policy. Nutritional Aspects of Cardiovascular Disease. Dept of Health: Report on Health & Social Subjects 46. HMSO 1994.

16 Muhlhauser I. Cigarette smoking and diabetes: an update. *Diabetic Medicine* 1994; **11**: 336–43.

17 Bulpitt CJ, Shaw KM, Hodes C, Bloom A. The symptom patterns of treated diabetic patients. *J Chron Dis* 1976; **29**: 571–83.

18 Gwilt DJ, Pentecost BL. The heart in diabetes in recent advances (2). In: Nattrass M (ed.), *Diabetes.* Churchill Livingstone 1986; 177–94.

19 Shaper AG, Perry IJ. Screening people with diabetes for risk of coronary heart disease in General Practice. *Practical Diabetes* 1994; **11**: 228–31.

20 Oswald GA, Yudkin JS. Hyperglycaemia following acute myocardial infarction;

the contributions of undiagnosed diabetes. *Diabetic Medicine* 1987; **4**: 68–70.
21 Bell DSH. Diabetic cardiomyopathy: A unique entity or a complication of coronary artery disease? *Diabetes Care* 1995; **18**: 708–14.
22 Jorgensen H, Nakayama H, Raaschou H, Olsen T. Effect of blood pressure and diabetes on stroke in progression. *Lancet* 1994; **344**: 156–9.
23 Orchard TJ, Strandness D. Assessment of peripheral vascular disease in diabetes. Report and recommendations of an International Workshop sponsored by the American Heart Association and the American Diabetes Association. *Diabetes Care* 1993; **16**: 1199–209.
24 Durrington PN. Prevention of macrovascular disease: Absolute Proof or Absolute Risk? *Diabetic Medicine*, 1995; **12**: 561–2.

9

Nursing Perspectives on Diabetic Complications

S. CRADOCK, A. TIER and J. WOOD

Department of Diabetes and Endocrinology,
Queen Alexandra Hospital, Portsmouth

INTRODUCTION

The prospect of potential complications as well as the presence of actual complications can be devastating for both the individual with diabetes and his or her family and friends. Professionals working in primary health care can often be in a unique position to offer help to such patients during their journey through life with diabetes.

This chapter will outline the issues, skills and considerations for primary health care professionals when assisting people with diabetes to prevent complications (by achievement of good blood glucose control and/or following a healthy lifestyle) or helping them when complications are present.

THE ROLE OF THE NURSE

All health care professionals have the ability to act as educators/motivators/supporters to the individual with diabetes, but often the nursing role can provide these skills in a more comprehensive way when working alongside the physician who is diagnosing and treating any potential complications that may arise.

Diabetic Complications. Edited by K. M. Shaw
© 1996 John Wiley & Sons Ltd

The *practice nurse* position is becoming such a role, but local experience suggests that time constraints still play a large part in missing opportunities to identify patients' fears and concerns. It is important to remember that even with only little time available, listening and practical advice can be as much a part of good diabetes care as adjusting medication. Often there is a need or attraction to concentrate on the medical screening aspects of diabetes care, when listening and helping the patient through his or her anxieties is as important. This is becoming increasingly important as some researchers are identifying a strong link between presence of complications and depression.

The *diabetes nurse specialist* role has developed over the past decade to varying degrees—most of these specialist nurses will work in close liaison with their primary care colleagues to ensure continuity of care for their patients. It is important that both diabetes nurse specialists and community nurses are aware of who is involved with the patient's care, so as not to waste the valuable time that is spent with the patient and thus greater use can be made of visits to clinics.

PREVENTIVE CARE

One of the main aspects of care of the patient with diabetes is that of trying to establish good glycaemic control and lifestyle behaviour, in order to prevent complications.

> If you give a man a fish he will have a single meal. If you teach him how to fish, he will eat all his life
>
> (Kuan-Tyer).

In order to help people develop the life skills required to prevent complications, we must all recognize that giving information should not just be seen as 'pot filling'[1]. It is so easy to believe that once you have given somebody information, he or she will readily act on this information, but recent health promotion studies have clearly shown this is not the case.

It is important to focus any teaching on to the patient's agenda—identifying the patient's needs and trying to motivate him or her towards turning the needs into the patient's 'wants'. Walker[2] suggested that meaningful education has to be learner centred—this can be time consuming, but is time well spent in the long term. Collaboration (not coercion) with the patient is essential in setting any education programme. Initially, the viewpoint of the patient must be sought—trying to find out what he or she already knows of potential complications.

VIGNETTE

James is a 28-year-old man who has recently developed IDDM. He is very concerned about the diagnosis, as his mother is now registered as visually handicapped—he admits to being worried that this will happen to him. But, what concerns him more are the memories he has of his mother having 'fits' when he was a child and is worried about the potential for this to happen to him, the effects of this on both of his young children and his job.

Any teaching should be suitable to the patient as an individual—this will require an indepth assessment of personal needs. The patient must be able to understand and follow the education programme in order to succeed and therefore the professional must regularly assess the progress of the patient's learning and pace the sessions/content accordingly. Often people will learn, experiment and consequently make mistakes. This is not to be seen as negative, but identified as normal and encouragement given to help people understand that we all make mistakes—the important thing is to learn from them. In fact, it is often the case that we learn best from our mistakes. Mistakes are frequently made with blood glucose monitoring testing, perhaps because initial teaching was inadequate. It is vital that people are confidently taught the correct way with no blame being attached. It is easy for health professionals to make some patients feel rather undermined.

Where to teach somebody can be important, although if the learner really wants to learn, the place is immaterial. But ideally, any environment that is conducive to learning will be relaxed and comfortable—the patient will 'want to come here'. While it is common in doctors' surgeries for desks to be sat behind and uniforms to be worn, there may be some times when this sort of environment is inappropriate. In saying this, one must remember again that it is the relationship with the patient that is most effective and often if the desk or uniform is a barrier, a skilled teacher can overcome this. Any teaching/learning environment needs to be set within an open and honest relationship, with health professionals recognizing that they may not know the answers to all the questions. But if they are purporting to be giving advice, then they should be as up to date as they possibly can be. The development of training programmes from local specialist diabetes teams can assist with these skills.

Any goals that may be jointly set with the patient must be achievable (within reach of the patient). This has been shown clearly to work, for example, in attaining some weight loss. If a target is set that is too great for somebody to achieve, or will take a long time to achieve, then it will be very difficult for that person to succeed in the short term. Goals should be set so that short-term success is obtainable. This success will motivate the patient to move on to further goal setting. At the end of each education session, it is vital that both parties evaluate what has happened so that progress can be monitored and achievements assessed. This is an ideal opportunity to allow for any repetition of information if necessary.

BEHAVIOUR CHANGE

When trying to encourage patients to make changes, it can be difficult to understand how well a patient is doing. A model of change[3] can be of help in understanding that people go through various stages in order to change and while relapse may occur, it should not be seen as failure:

- *Pre-contemplation*. The person is not interested in changing a 'risky' lifestyle. He or she may be unaware of the risks being run.

- *Contemplation*. Once aware of potential risks, an individual may start to think about making changes.

- *Action*. When the possible benefits of change are seen, the individual prepares for change, often needing extra skills and support. The initial changes tend to need positive decisions. Clear goals and achievable plans are necessary for success in this stage.

- *Maintaining change*. Once changes are made, the individual has to adjust to a new behaviour. Occasionally, maintaining this new behaviour is difficult, requiring constant support to avoid 'relapse'.

- *Relapsing*. Relapse is normal and should not be seen as a failing (for patient or helper). Assistance can then be provided to move into the contemplative stage.

This model has been adapted locally for use with people who have diabetes, using a 'five phase' structure. During each phase the individual will go through the 'change process'. Once maintaining changes and prepared to make further changes, a person will progress to the next phase.

GIVING OF INFORMATION/BREAKING BAD NEWS

It's not what you say, but the way you say it.

Health professionals often are a bit wary of telling patients about the potential of complications or the fact that the patient is showing signs of the development of same. It is frequently hard to know how much a patient should be told about the complications of diabetes and this is a question that is often asked of specialist teams. If all potential problems were explained to people with diabetes, they might give up from the start. On the other hand, can we or should we withhold information? Will the patient feel a full sense of security, and could health professionals be blamed when things start to go wrong?

It is apparent therefore that patients do need to know something about the complications of diabetes. Hindley[4] states that we are not doing people with diabetes any favours by hiding the facts from them, which suggests that all health professionals have a level of accountability to their patients and this should be borne in mind when considering the amount of information given. One point to remember is that we may not be the only people that are giving that person information—the media, diabetic leaflets, library books, friends and relatives are all providers of information, which can sometimes be conflicting. We must help people to understand how to interpret various messages that they may be given and thus make informed choices about their care, but one difficulty is that the facts seem to be constantly changing. Some people reading this book will have learnt about the potential reduction in some complications, but if health professionals have worked in the health care industry for a long time, they may still have memories of patients commonly being admitted with severe complications. The environment in which a professional works will also influence his or her attitude and potential knowledge/advice about diabetic complications.

VIGNETTE

Albert is a 70-year-old man who has had non-insulin-dependent diabetes for years. He had a left below-knee amputation a year ago. With only input from his GP, Albert describes himself as 'having had no education'. He cares for his demented wife, who is doubly incontinent. He is quoted as saying 'I had no idea I could influence what was happening to me. My GP kept saying my diabetes was poorly controlled, but I felt that it was in his hands. Of course I would have made changes if I knew what to change.' Albert is now wheelchair bound and struggling to care for his wife, feeling let down by someone—his GP—whom he trusted. This sort of patient can be very difficult to motivate towards further changes to protect his future health.

All professionals must remember that they have a duty to provide correct appropriate information. Our understanding of complications is constantly changing and we must keep up to date if we are putting ourselves into a position to provide information. We must then listen to the effect of the information that we have given to the patient and correct any mis-understanding that may have occurred. While we may think we have clearly stated a fact, often another person will hear what we have said in a different way. When giving information regarding complications, it is important to assess what the patient already has heard, or assumed about complications, before building on that knowledge.

VIGNETTE

Peter is a 58-year-old man, who has had non-insulin-dependent diabetes for 20 years and has been on insulin therapy for the last 10 years. Since his diagnosis, he has followed a very strict diet (having only one potato with each meal, and never touching alcohol or sweet foods). He believes that he will become blind very shortly as the same occurred to his mother prior to her death a number of years ago. He has no evidence of developing retinopathy—indeed, after 30 years of diabetes, he has only occasional background retinopathy. He has not had the benefit of current knowledge and information regarding both the development and treatment of retinopathy, as well as the greater potential for good blood glucose control in recent years since the advent of blood glucose monitoring and better insulin regimens.

COMMUNICATION AND GIVING OF INFORMATION

The skills required by any health professional for informational care are the same skills that are used in the counselling approach:

1. *Open questions*. These allow the patient to talk, indeed encourage the patient to talk. Open questions are those that cannot be answered with a yes or no (these are described as closed questions).

2. *Active listening*. This is the opposite to passive listening where the listener is just simply taking in what is being said. Active listeners constantly respond to what is being said to them by the patient—this enables a very clear picture to be built up by the professional on what the patient is thinking and feeling. It also allows any misunderstanding on the professional's part to be checked with the patient, so that corrections can be made.

3. *Reflection*. In their own words, professionals pick up on what the patient has said showing their understanding of the situation and in doing so give the patient opportunity to explore/express his or her feelings further.

4. *Unconditional positive regard*. If the health professional is wanting to help the patient move forward in the management of his or her health,

then there is great need for a non-judgemental approach and attitude—this would include an acceptance of present behaviour.

Patients obviously differ in the way that they deal with situations. Patient-centred approaches leave no room for predetermined education plans or routinely applied checklists—which often appear to help the professional, but frequently do not benefit the patient. Another advantage of using a patient-focused or patient-centred approach is that it tends to lead to enhanced motivation.

DIABETES CONTROL AND COMPLICATIONS TRIAL/ST VINCENT'S DECLARATION

The Diabetes Control and Complications Trial (DCCT 1993)[5] demonstrated quite clearly that good glycaemic control helps to prevent or delay the onset of complications and the St Vincent's Declaration (1992)[6] starts to give us some standards on which to base our care in order to reduce the impact of these complications.

With any research study, as in the DCCT, health professionals must be fully aware of the nature of the study before exalting its results. In order to achieve good control in this long-term study, it required a lot of time and hard work on both the patients'/professionals' part as well as a large financial investment. At the moment, most health professionals are not in a position to provide such care. Also the patients were recruited by advertisements in local newspapers and were therefore a fairly self-selected group. A number of the patients had to be free of complications to enter one part of the study, and this probably put them into a lower risk group initially.

It is important not to use such studies as a stick to wield over the patient, but rather as a carrot to encourage change.

Most studies looking at the development of complications will give us an idea of the percentage of people who are likely to get complications, and more recently the risk factors that may potentially put somebody at risk of those complications. Unfortunately, we are still not in a position to be able to predict at the onset of diabetes those that are at greater risk. It can be very difficult for both the health care professional and the patient if good control is not achieved, as both can feel guilty. An understanding of the spectrum of diabetes care and management by patients is vital as one patient's experience may not be the same as another's—there will always be a patient that has managed to follow a less than healthy diet, who has reached a good age without complications, as there will always be the person that has smoked cigarettes for 50 years and has escaped lung cancer.

SELF-CARE

The aim of the educational approach in diabetes is to encourage patients to manage their own diabetes, by encouraging development of skills to problem solve and the ability to select additional support from health care professionals as they require it. Teaching somebody something is not just showing him or her what to do—it is important to check that the person has learnt from the teaching and knows what to do with what has been learnt. For example, it is technically reasonable to show somebody how to monitor blood glucose, but it will be a total waste of time unless the patient also knows why he or she should do it, and how to use the information that the blood tests are providing.

> Jim (*out walking his dog Spot*) says to his friend Bob: 'I taught Spot how to whistle'.
> Bob (*bending and listening for Spot to whistle*): 'I don't hear him whistling'.
> Jim: 'I said I **taught** him, I didn't say he'd **learnt** it'.

Recent small studies have shown clearly that people are more likely to maintain such testing if they are using it to improve their diabetic control. This will be true of any lifestyle skills, e.g. giving up smoking, reducing fat in the diet. People need to know why they need to do it and some appropriate ways of how to actually change their lifestyle. Patients should feel and know that they are making an informed choice to change their lifestyle if they so wish. There are very few patients around who will do as they are told just because they have been told to.

VIGNETTE

David is a 45-year-old man, who has had insulin-dependent diabetes for 15 years. He has been coming regularly for annual screening and in the last few years it has been clear that his albumin:creatinine ratio is rising—putting him at risk from nephropathy. It was suggested by the medical practitioner that he should take some Captopril tablets as a protective measure for the kidneys (see Chapter 2). He refused to do this and walked away from the clinic quite despondent. Fortunately, the medical practitioner referred him to the nurse specialist, who spent some time with David trying to understand his frustrations and for him to explain why he was not prepared to accept the treatment. It transpired that he did not understand why he should take a tablet, when he felt so well and there was no demonstrable medical problem. It also became clear that David was 'struggling' generally with his diabetes control, trying to reduce his carbohydrate intake in order to lower his blood sugars. He had not had opportunity for a dietary review in the past 10 years and was still following carbohydrate restriction! By altering his diet, reducing the potential for hypoglycaemia, enabling him to increase his insulin and reduce his blood glucose level appropriately, he also felt confident to make the decision to start taking Captopril.

The traditional health professional role is very different to that of patient empowerment. The word empowerment is a much maligned word in recent years and still some health professionals are uncertain of how to manage an empowering relationship with their patient[7]. Using an empowering approach stops the need for the use of the word 'compliance', which implies that people are doing what they are told. The use of 'self-care' or 'self-management' may be a better choice of phrase. It has been suggested that in actual fact non-compliance is quite common and is normal. If one considers this on a wider basis, then it would be a very strange society in which we lived if everyone did as they were told by somebody else. Human beings will tend to behave as others want them to behave only if they recognize the value of doing so, but unfortunately in diabetes, disregarding medical advice may lead to complications and it can be hard for health professionals not to be judgemental and consider even quietly in their own mind the phrase 'I told you so'.

VIGNETTE

Katharine is a young woman, who has had diabetes for about 12 years. She has had numerous 'social' issues throughout her life that have seemed to get in the way of her achieving 'good control'. In more recent years her problems have subsided, but she has still found it quite difficult to get 'good control' and this has resulted in long-term high blood glucose levels. In recent months she became pregnant, which required radical changes in her lifestyle but these changes were easy for Katharine to adopt now that she was motivated by the potential birth of a healthy baby. Within one month her HbA1C had reduced from 18% to 8%. Sadly, however, the problems of this change led to worsened eye damage requiring laser treatment. There was a need for her baby to be induced at 32 weeks of pregnancy. Katharine is now beginning to feel cheated by working hard at making changes—her health professionals may also feel somewhat cheated and confused.

The relationship we develop with our patients who have diabetes may well be long term. It is helpful to both parties to establish a better grounding of the relationship so that honesty and truth become paramount. This will lead, hopefully, to an increased desire by the patient, to make the changes as requested, but also an increased acceptance by the health professional of whatever changes, be they none or just a few, are made by the patient.

Self-care or self-management of diabetes will be affected quite strongly by stressful situations, which in today's world are very difficult to avoid. Before any success is going to be achieved by the patient or the health professional, some recognition of these situations is necessary and, if possible, some means of assisting in the reduction of the effect of them.

For example, emotional trauma from a recent divorce or death of a friend or relative, will obstruct the patient from achieving his or her true potential in health care changes.

MOTIVATION—'WHAT TURNS PEOPLE ON'

Motivational studies have shown that the best results are achieved by encouragement. In all walks of life the 'halo effect' is dominant[8]. If we are successful, then we become more successful. If, however, we feel a failure, we will more likely become a failure. Threatening people with future possible complications will not necessarily lead to compliance. Moreover, the patient can easily be led to feel inadequate or pessimistic. As health professionals we must try and achieve a happy balance, being able to give honest optimistic options to all patients, young and old.

It is useful to avoid terms such as 'poor control', 'bad diet' or 'non-compliance'. Blaming or labelling patients can be damaging to their self-esteem. Or, if it is difficult to change the words we use, we must be very aware of the way in which we are using these phrases—it may be difficult to get rid of the term 'poor control' but we must be certain that the patient is not completely blaming himself or herself for that poor control.

All health professionals will have met patients who they know are trying their best to achieve their potential in diabetes care management, but still have diabetes that is difficult to control—even if it is related to their character/personality. It may be necessary to seek help of third parties (dietitians, psychologists, etc.) in order to help with the root cause of some problems.

As human beings, we all have the potential to change whatever in our life we would like to, but what really motivates us comes from within and sustained change in behaviour has to be generated from internal motivation. Most health professionals, by providing advice and information, will at best be providing extrinsic motivational potential, i.e. putting the need to change on a short-term basis to please others. How often have we met people who at the start of their diagnosis of diabetes have made major changes in their life, but within a year or so those changes have relapsed and they are perhaps not following the best diet or lifestyle that they had originally hoped that they would (see Figure 9.1). This is a clear case of extrinsic motivation (professional input and possibly symptoms of the disease) affecting behaviour. As soon as professional support is withdrawn or the person is feeling better, it is easy to lapse. One of the difficulties with diabetes specifically is that people can remain very well in the short term with blood sugars running

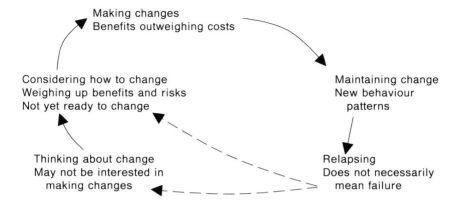

Figure 9.1. The process of change. (Adapted from reference 3)

between 10 and 13 mmol/l—yet it is quite clear that this level of blood glucose control can cause complications in some people.

The literature suggests that education programmes alone will increase knowledge about diabetes self-management, but will only improve gly-caemic control in the short term, if at all. A clear example of this is that doctors and nurses are well aware of the dangers of smoking, but many continue to do so. Why should the non-compliant patient be any different? It is not enough to say, 'But they must change their behaviour. They have diabetes and could run into problems.' It can be difficult for people with diabetes to associate short-term control with the effect of long-term com-plications. Diabetes is a silent disease—slowly but surely damaging tissues over a period of time.

> **VIGNETTE**
>
> Jenny knew that she could go blind with diabetes, but had not linked this with the interest shown by her doctors in her blood glucose levels. She always felt all right— no symptoms of thirst or polyuria, which she had thought meant her diabetes was out of control. She had not seen the connection, therefore did not attend the majority of clinic appointments, as she disliked seeing other patients with white sticks and amputations.

Another aspect of reduced self-management in patients may be something to do with the environment in which we see them. The St Vincent guide-lines for encouraging well-being suggest that we should identify dis-satisfactions with aspects of the service that we provide—how often have we been put off going to a shop in the high street because of the way that the last shop assistant dealt with us? It may have only been an off day for that person, but it made us think that the whole shop was tainted with the same attitude. Our diabetes centres, primary health care diabetic clinics, GP surgeries may cause some difficulties with some patients. If we really are committed to helping people improve their control, perhaps we have to think about changing the environment in which we are providing our service in order that they attend our appointments. It is not enough for health professionals to emphasize their value, patients also must see them as valuable to them. It is not suggested that we tailor our service to meet the needs of every individual—this would be impossible given the present economic restraints—but as we know that those patients who do not attend diabetic clinics are more likely to be those that develop complications, should we not be considering some changes? It may be that simply the structure of the clinic is difficult for some patients to cope with.

We should perhaps consider also that achieving perfect health is not the ultimate gain for all human beings. We are constantly told that it should be the ideal, especially as it will reduce the financial burden on the state by people looking after their own health more effectively, but health professionals are constantly aware of people whose main aim in life is not to do so. Perhaps as health professionals we would be more effective in helping people change if we tried to see a view of the world from their perspective—if nothing else, it would give us an opportunity to see whether there are any potential motivating factors in their perspective rather than our perspective.

COMMUNICATION

As we are seeking good control and effective lifestyle changes in our patients, all health professionals need to be communicating effectively with each other, as well as with their patients. We all need to be clear about each other's priorities and concerns. Breakdown in communications can quickly lead to problems—with all involved putting up natural defences or coping mechanisms. Health carers in an ideal world would be saying the same things—and in close knit teams this is quite reasonable to expect—but as mentioned before, people with diabetes will get information about diabetes from all sorts of areas. Perhaps a role for health professionals is to help patients be aware of the different information that they may acquire.

An increasing communication problem is that of cultural language differences (for example, the Asian population). This may cause problems and often leads to a 'second class' service. Inexperience of a culture can cause problems for health professionals. Those working in areas with few ethnic minorities may be more likely to provide a two-tier system, as they have little experience of the needs of such cultures. The increasingly wide-spread use of translators is seen to be very helpful, as they not only trans-late the language but help health professionals understand the culture. All of this will require increased knowledge and understanding on the part of the professional and again environmental systems may need to change.

Communication problems can also occur within families, especially where children have been diagnosed at a young age and the parents have naturally taken control of the diabetes in the early years. It is quite evident that when children become adolescents, with the natural rebelliousness of teenagers, they suddenly realize the impact that their diabetes is having on their lives and will respond to this knowledge in different ways. If parents have perhaps controlled the diabetes quite tightly, all involved will become frustrated when there is a loss of control during adolescent years, which may be a result of teenagers experimenting with the diabetes that they now regard as their own. Health professionals will need to support parents as well as the adolescents through this stage. Parents may under-stand the future potential for complications and may well become terrified of the sudden loss of blood glucose control, and the potential risk on their children's health in the near future.

SCREENING FOR COMPLICATIONS

There is a shared responsibility for the screening of complications, both between primary and secondary health care and between nursing and medical professions. Who does what with regards to screening the patients in annual review will vary depending on the interest and roles within each surgery. Clearly though the practice nurse has a major role in ensuring that the patient is being screened, that recall systems are effective and possibly what is happening to those results when screened. Generally, the aim is for nurses and doctors to work in partnership to ensure nobody slips through any loopholes in the local health care system.

PATIENT ASSESSMENT

When seeing any patient with diabetes, it is worth having a checklist of physical aspects of their health to assess. This can help with the detailed examination that may be undertaken by the physician. Family history of diabetes and complications will help the professional understand two things: firstly, whether there is an increased likelihood of complications occurring in this patient; and, secondly, whether there will be any potential underlying fears of complications. The duration of diabetes in any patient will give a clue as to the likelihood of complications. For those people with insulin-dependent diabetes of less than five years' duration the presence of complications is unlikely, so the emphasis should be on management of control rather than seeking out complications. In somebody with insulin-dependent diabetes who has been diagnosed for longer than 5 years, the dual approach is required. In a patient who has had diabetes for 30 or more years, whatever the patient has been achieving during his or her life with diabetes is suggested to have been successful, although the emphasis on reasonable control should not necessarily be relaxed—this will depend on age and general health.

In a patient with non-insulin-dependent diabetes, the emphasis on complication screening will start from diagnosis, as it is recognized that some of these patients may well have had undiagnosed diabetes for a number of years, and therefore the ravages of poor control and lipid disorders may already be taking their toll. Assessment of diabetic control will also give clues as to potential complications—it is clear that people who run average blood glucose levels below 10 mmol/l are less at risk of developing complications. This control should be sustained, but as yet we have no information as to whether short bursts of poor control amongst generally good control is damaging. Abnormal blood lipid levels will also suggest a potential risk for macrovascular disease and increased emphasis should be placed on lifestyle changes (diet, exercise, smoking).

Weight changes and obesity will provide information on potential risk of complications. It is clearly demonstrated that obesity is a risk factor contributing towards macrovascular disease. Loss of weight in an insulin-dependent or non-insulin-dependent patient may signify worsening diabetic control (in the absence of dieting) and should be noted and acted on quickly. Weight gain in an insulin-dependent patient may suggest too much insulin and while the blood glucose control is showing high sugars, there may be times when low blood sugars are present but not being monitored—a reduction in insulin may help both problems.

Activity levels should be assessed and greater effort put into encouraging those at risk to increase their level of activity. It is important for health professionals not to expect too much of their patients (in the same way they would not expect too much of themselves!). Evidence suggests that just an increased walking level during the day can offer some health gain.

Urine testing will give information regarding prevailing blood glucose control in the hours previous to the consultation, but there is clear evidence that this only gives a suggestion of control rather than quantifiable results. Proteinuria must be recorded and checked again as this could be a measure of worsening renal function. More recently, there is evidence to suggest the testing of microalbuminuria by various methods (see Chapter 2). Local protocols will govern the types of patient to be tested and the action on results of tests. In any case, any presence of proteinuria in the diabetic patient should be treated with potential seriousness.

A foot assessment can act as an educational tool to the patient, but also give the health professional some information on the potential foot complications of diabetes. By being aware of the 'normal' foot, all nurses can potentially identify the 'at risk' foot (see Chapter 7).

When to assess will vary. Some teams will involve patients in regular screening opportunities, others will use opportunities as they arise, rather than established screening programmes. It is important to ensure that whatever system is in use, a patient is getting some screening each year. Any opportunity to assess a patient can offer some gain, so whenever a patient is in a GP surgery or in hospital, there is an opportunity to provide advice and reinforcing information. Often people will know of the areas of their life that they need to change, e.g. smoking and diet, and will not need constant reminding of the need to change—what they may need help with is how to effect the change for themselves.

Psychological assessment is important as it may well uncover depression, which may hinder the progress of the individual to improve self-care.

VIGNETTE

John has peripheral neuropathy and reduced circulation. He has been in a system of regular follow-up by both primary and secondary care teams. He has also had advice on numerous occasions about taking care of his feet from his podiatrist. All of this though, did not prevent an ulcer occurring on one of his toes—noticed not by John, but by the podiatrist as John's sock was removed to attend to a previous ulcer. Despite all the information and teaching that John had been given—it appeared that the health professionals had overlooked the fact that John may not have changed his behaviour as a result of knowledge.

ESTABLISHED COMPLICATIONS

Once complications have 'set in' it is important that the health professionals do not give up on the patient, i.e. remove the emphasis on good control, etc. We now have clear evidence that any improvement of control in patients with established complications can halt the deterioration of such complications. The patient will also need even more support than has been given before. Some health care systems may prevent this—some tertiary care systems (e.g. renal units) may take over the complete management of the patient, but will only be tackling things from their specialist perspective and less emphasis will be given to general diabetes care. Health care teams should try and ensure that the chances of this happening are minimal.

CONCLUSION

The complications of diabetes and their prevention should be in the forefront of any health professional's mind when meeting with such patients. But, while good control and healthy lifestyles are important, they will not be achieved without the individual experiencing some quality of life. In order for us to help people with diabetes achieve both, we must consider the prevention and management of complications with a non-judgemental, optimistic and knowledgeable approach, remembering that the patients themselves will be making the final decisions about their care. The ideal approach is one of the team working in a collaborative way with the patient.

REFERENCES

1 Coles CR. Diabetes education: Letting the patient into the picture. *Practical Diabetes* 1990; **7**: 110–12.
2 Walker R. Education: principles and practice. *Diabetic Nursing* 1991; **2**(3): 4–7.
3 Prochaska JO, Diclemente CC. Towards a comprehensive model of change. In: Miller WR, Heather N (eds), *Treating Addictive Behaviours, Processes of Change*. New York: Plenum, 1986.
4 Hindley P. 'Back to Basics'—British Diabetic Association, Diabetes Newsline, Sept (report of talk given PSS Bournemouth, May 1987).
5 DCCT Diabetes Control and Complications Trial Research Group. The effect of intensive diabetes treatment on the development and progression of long-term complications in insulin dependent diabetes mellitus. *N Engl J Med* 1993; **329**: 977–86.
6 St Vincent, Krans HMJ, Porta M, Keen H. *Diabetes Care and Research in Europe*. The St Vincent Declaration Action Programme, World Health Organization, 1992.
7 Brown FJ. The role of counselling in diabetes care. *Practical Diabetes* 1988; **5**(4): 174–5.
8 Child D. *Psychology and the Teacher*. London: Holt, Rinehart & Winston, 1981.

Index

Note: Page numbers in *italic* refer to figures and/or tables

Index compiled by Caroline Sheard